The Kidney Donor's Journey:

100 Questions I Asked Before Donating My Kidney

Ari Sytner

The Kidney Donor's Journey: 100 Questions I Asked Before Donating My Kidney

ISBN: 978-0-9981984-0-8

Dedication

Dedicated to my dear grandparents, of blessed memory. Without knowing it, their influence on shaping my life was truly profound.

I hope to one day be such a grandparent.

Table of Contents

Chapter 2:
The Testing Process 30

Chapter 3:
Weighing The Risks & Making a Decision 60

Chapter 4.
The Fear of Telling Other People

Chapter 5:
The Surgery 101

Chapter 6:
Recovering in the Hospital....... 126

Chapter 7:
Recovering at Home 142

Chapter 8:
The Rest of My Life............ 158

Chapter 9:
Conclusion 170

Chapter 10:
Testimonials 179

Acknowledgments

Life is a canvas and the people we encounter become our brushstrokes. This book captures a picture of my incredible journey through kidney donation. It is an experience I was only blessed to have because of the range of very special people I have encountered throughout my life. Thus, when I think about my kidney donation, it is not a deed that I alone can ever take credit for in a vacuum. For it was not me alone who donated my kidney, but it was a team effort. It was the result of countless special people in my life who contributed to, inspired, supported and guided me through this journey.

First and foremost, I am eternally grateful to my incredible wife, Chana, whose wisdom, love and constant support made this experience, and everything else I have ever accomplished, entirely possible. I am truly appreciative, and continually in awe of all that Chana is and does, not only for our family, but for our community and the world around us. In addition, as you will read in this book, it was my four unbelievably amazing kids, Reuven, Meyer, Akiva and Aliza who all played critical roles in inspiring me to donate my kidney. Additionally, I owe everything I am to my father and mother for a lifetime of love, support, nurturing and encouragement. Furthermore, the love I received from grandparents, who constantly showered me with examples of love and kindness, helped shape me into a person who lives each day to enrich the lives of others. I also could not ask for better siblings, who serve as constant role models for performing deeds of kindness, always with humility and always with a smile. Their influence upon me has been beyond transformative.

I cannot imagine what my life would look like without the rabbis, teachers, mentors and friends who have truly molded me in countless ways. Yet, perhaps the most impactful relationships over the years have been my many students and congregants, who have always inspired me, and for whom I am eternally grateful. This includes, but is not limited to all our dear friends in Charleston, South Carolina, who lovingly supported our family through this journey, and the Zucker family, who never cease to amaze me with their own shining examples of kindness and promoting the Jewish value of Tikkun Olam (doing everything one can do to help improve the world).

The kidney journey itself could not have happened without the incredible patience, support and encouragement of Chaya Lipschutz of Kidney Mitzvah; Sam Waldman, Pat McDonough, Dr. Stuart Greenstein; and the staff at Montefiore Medical Center. Additionally, I extend a special token of appreciation to the wonderful people of Renewal for all of their ongoing work to support hundreds of altruistic kidney donations, as well as the countless non-profit organizations dedicated to helping support those with kidney disease.

Writing this book has been a journey unto itself, and there are countless people that have been incredibly supportive with the publishing, editing, marketing, formatting, design and distribution of the book. I owe a special debt of gratitude to the hundreds of people from around the world who have generously contributed to and supported this endeavor. Additionally, I am indebted to a number of very talented and passionate people for going well above and beyond to help me reach my publishing goals. This includes, Suzi Day, Robyn Stevens, Harvey Mysel, Dr. Virginia Irwin-Scott, Dr. Scherly Leon, Valen Keefer, and Dr. Sigrid Fry-Revere.

However, the single most instrumental person who enabled this journey to become a reality, is Ronit (pronounced *row-neat*), my dear, precious, beloved kidney recipient. While I would have been happy to give my kidney to anyone, I could not have asked for a better and more kind-hearted person to love and welcome my kidney into its new home. Together with her three amazing kids, Dana, Lilach and Barr, Ronit Havivi has a zest for life that is a true inspiration!

Finally, I humbly express my profound appreciation to God. Not only have I felt Divine guidance throughout the entire kidney donation process - as everything fell so smoothly into place - but I have felt that guidance at every stage of my life. On a daily basis, through God's benevolence, I have been blessed to experience firsthand what absolute kindness feels like. I could not have asked for a greater role model to demonstrate this value to me, and inspire me to pay forward to others, what I have undeservedly been so blessed to receive.

Introduction

I strongly believe in the human spirit and the unlimited capacity of people to be givers. Yet, on a daily basis, each person is confronted with numerous opportunities, great and small, to express their selflessness. Surprisingly, however, only some people "give," while others do not. As a kidney donor, I have often wondered about this distinction. If there are, in fact, billions of extra kidneys in the world, and people are generally kind-hearted, why do more people not come forward to offer this incredible gift of life to others?

It is with all my heart that I believe that the lack of kidney donors in the world is not due to lack of compassion or caring for our fellow. Rather, I believe it is due to a lack of awareness and understanding about the process of kidney donation. This belief led me to realize that a comprehensive book was necessary to outline the altruistic donor's personal experience, so that others can be given an insider's view of every aspect, question and struggle of the journey.

However, despite my deep desire to write this book in an effort to help those awaiting a kidney donation, I constantly hesitated. In fact, I find it quite uncomfortable to author these pages, as I do not enjoy speaking about my kidney donation, nor drawing attention to myself, as if I were a hero of sorts. I am simply an ordinary person who saw someone in need and offered to help.

However, despite not wanting to draw attention to my deeply personal journey, after seeing how my kidney was able to so drastically change the life of, not only the recipient, but the entire family, I felt compelled to share my journey in the hopes of educating and inspiring others to learn, ask, research and explore this topic.

When I first began my journey of exploring kidney donation, I was light-years away from ever going through with it. I was merely intrigued and curious. I had dozens of questions that I wished to ask. Yet, when I began to scour the Internet, I found an abundance of confusing information (and sometimes misinformation). Most of the websites I found offered a very basic overview of kidney donation, all from the lens of the hospitals and doctors. My first frustration was that I did not want to learn about the topic from the very people who were promoting it. I was skeptical of hospitals trying to convince me that kidney donation was perfectly safe. After all, as for-profit institutions, I felt that they were biased. Moreover, on every one of their websites I encountered an inevitable call to action. In other words, "here is some basic information about kidney donation, but give us your phone number and we will call you to setup an appointment and discuss it further." And all I could think was, "Slow down!"

At that early stage, I was not ready for action, I was simply filled with curiosity to know whether it was a topic that I wished to explore further. There was a huge gap between being merely curious and visiting the local transplant hospital.

Considering the chasm that existed between curiosity and action, I realized that most donors would never have an accessible roadmap to help guide them through the process. That is why I wrote this book, which aims to serve as a bridge to educate and empower ordinary people to see a more complete picture of the kidney donation roadmap, all through the lens of my own experience and journey.

Since I am not a doctor or medical professional, this book should not serve as medical advice. Rather, I urge each person to follow my example and ask all questions to one's own doctors and medical professionals. The perspective throughout this book is unique, as I detail not only the process of my own exploration, but my personal reactions and feelings - sharing the private, familial and emotional components to this journey. This book serves as a roadmap to help understand what a potential donor might think, feel and struggle with, as he or she embarks upon this incredible exploration.

Considering my own insecurities over whether or not to break my silence and speak up, I recently conducted an online poll, asking whether kidney donors should remain quiet about their donation, or share it with others. I was shocked at the response, wherein a large majority of people felt that kidney donation was a private act and need not be shared with others. Some viewed it as if speaking up was a form of bragging. Nevertheless, despite public sentiments and remaining quiet for several years, I forced myself to write this book, feeling compelled to break my own silence to help those in need. For if I had another kidney to give, I would gladly do so. Yet, since I have already done my part in donating, all I can still do is share my own story with others in the hopes of advocating for those in need.

It was during my journey that I realized that people awaiting a kidney have an impossible question to ask. They are forced to turn to a friend, neighbor or family member and literally ask for a piece of their body. The amount of guilt and shame associated with that question can be painful and crippling, preventing one from getting life-saving help. Therefore, by creating this book, I aim to empower kidney patients with an easier, more palatable question. Instead of asking whether someone would consider donating a kidney, they can now ask, "would you consider reading a book?" Through these pages, one gains an insider's perspective, without making any commitment, to enable them to know whether or not they wish to begin their own journey. However, as my journey demonstrates, the decision is not merely a yes or no question to be answered. It is a series of personal, ethical and existential struggles and contradictions that must be reconciled. Ultimately, through this process one's heart, mind and soul can undergo a deeply transformational experience.

I have specifically written this book in a question/answer format to empower readers to approach this topic with great skepticism. This is not a process to jump into blindly, but one which requires questions to be asked at every turn. *This book is not intended to convince people to donate a kidney.* It aims to raise awareness about a very serious problem affecting millions of people worldwide. By mapping out the process I went through, the book creates a framework that can help others tackle the many questions that must be asked. It reflects the exploration of how human life is valued, and to what extent one might go to preserve and save a life. The decision to donate a kidney is not one to be taken lightly. It is something which is done over time and only through finding answers to a wide range of questions. Ultimately, the questions, answers and stories that are documented in these pages are an expression of my own personal struggles at each turn in the process.

The book neatly breaks down the journey into the stages of my exploration, including the steps I took to learn about kidney donation; the testing process; the surgery; the recovery; and how this one act would impact the rest of my life. Simply by taking the time to read this book, you are taking action to help make a difference in the lives of millions of kidney patients who wait, long, hope and pray for someone like you to come along and champion the cause of kidney donation.

Chapter 1.
Starting the Journey

1. Why would I consider kidney donation?

The truth is, when I began this journey, kidney donation was not something I had any connection to. I did not know anyone in renal failure, nor did I respond to a call to be tested for donation. In fact, it was all quite out of the blue and was not something I had ever considered.

By way of appreciating some context, it is worthwhile to note that I am generally a very risk-averse person. I am not a thrill-seeker. I don't do extreme sports, and I despise roller coaster rides. In fact, before this journey began, I had never even donated blood! Thus, by many accounts, as a husband and father of four children, I would be considered the last person on earth that you one would expect to donate a kidney. For most people who begin to explore kidney donation, they do so in response to someone they know who is in need of a transplant and taps them on the shoulder, introducing them to this entirely new world. However, my story was quite different.

For a number of years, I had the pleasure of serving as the rabbi of a beautiful congregation in the South. In addition to leading prayer services, tending to the pastoral needs of the congregation and running a host of educational programs, I was always on the lookout for new and exciting topics to teach. In the hopes of trying to attract a larger crowd eager to learn about a cutting-edge topic, I decided to launch an educational series on medical ethics. As I prepared and taught numerous lessons about stem cells, brain death and organ donation, I learned a great deal about these subjects. I highlighted to my students the importance and value of saving and preserving human life, in contrast with the challenges of pushing medical and ethical boundaries. I challenged my students with thought-provoking questions, such as: How much risk should be taken by one human life, both morally and ethically, in order to save another? Is the value of someone else's life worth more than my own? Do I have the right to jeopardize my own wellbeing for that of another? Should saving a life differ if it is a young child versus an older adult? Does it change the ethics of the debate if life were only to be extended for a short period of time?

For weeks, these issues were raised, unpacked and explored, as we delved deeply into them. By the time the course was all over, I had presented many layers of ethical dilemmas associated with kidney donation. I recall standing before my congregation and concluding the lesson by explaining what a wonderful

Mitzvah (a good deed) it was to donate a kidney in order to save a life.

However, after I went home that night, I distinctly remember feeling like a complete hypocrite! There I was, telling others to consider donating a kidney, but it was not something I would ever do. That was the very moment that really began the journey for me. Let me be clear, however, that it was not the moment I decided to donate a kidney, rather it was then I decided to challenge myself to at least explore the topic more carefully and learn how kidney donation might fit into my life. Upon deeper reflection, I came to the conclusion that not donating a kidney was certainly a viable option for me. However, if I was not going to donate a kidney, it would only be after further research and a conscious choice, rather than simply looking away from the issue and ignoring the suffering of others around me.

My starting point for this journey was one of compassion, combined with my desire to at least ask myself what I could do to help the lives of people in need.

2. What is the value of a human life?

Often people are surprised to learn that I am a kidney donor. The first question they ask me is, "Really? Who did you donate to, a relative or a friend?"

The answer is, neither. I donated my kidney to a total stranger.

Then follows, the second question, which almost all people think, but only some ask, "wow, are you crazy?!"

The truth is that one has to be just a little bit "crazy" to consider kidney donation. However, not any "crazier" than those who become firefighters, police officers, or join the military.

Considering the fact that prior to this journey I had never met or known a kidney donor, nor did I recall ever knowing anyone who needed an organ transplant, it seemed quite far-fetched that I would ever become a donor. What, then, compelled me to do something, which most people would consider to be so extreme?

Imagine if you saw a child drowning in a lake, would you stand by and just watch? Certainly most people, without even thinking or hesitating, would jump in and attempt to save a life - even at personal risk. Why? Because we all share a common value for life.

Ironically, if the scenario were changed and one was asked to save a life by donating a kidney, most people would hesitate.

If both scenarios involve saving a life, why might a person have such drastically different responses to two very similar scenarios?

Firstly, with kidney donation, unlike the drowning victim, there is a physical buffer which allows us to simply look away. As a society, we are aware that there are millions of people who are in need of kidney donations. Intellectually, we know they exist and we know they are dying. However, since we do not observe their suffering, or the urgency of their plight, nor do we necessarily know who they are, we can more easily return to our routine without giving it much further thought. Whereas in the case of a person drowning, looking away and returning to regular life is simply not an option, because we directly observe their suffering and experience the urgency.

But, like most people, when I first considered the thought of kidney donation, my mind immediately raced towards dreaded fears of surgery, needles and pain. However, I soon realized that the surgery is not the proper starting point - there is plenty of time to think about, research, and explore it later. The first step is to spend time pondering the value of life and the ability that one person has to help another in need.

When I first learned that there are people who are tethered for hours each day to a dialysis machine, unable to work or enjoy their lives or their children, in constant fear and mental anguish over whether they will live or die, I was motivated enough to look in the mirror and ask what I can do to help. While, early on I was unable to commit to donating a kidney, I became fascinated with the notion that I have the ability to save someone's life.

I knew that with my kidney I was holding the key to another person's salvation. The more I thought about it, the more I realized that when in utero, being formed as a healthy fetus, I was given two perfect kidneys, although I only needed one to survive. I knew that I had taken these kidneys with me throughout my life and I would ultimately one day leave this world. At that time, I would be buried with two perfect kidneys, while someone out there could have been given a second chance at life, if only I had shared one of those precious gifts that were given to me.

When this powerful idea becomes the starting point for the journey, it creates perspective. One cannot put all the surgical risks on one side of the scale, without first determining the value and weight of what will be placed on the other side of the scale. Once a person recognizes that it is life itself which hangs in the balance, then one can question what would outweigh it on the other side.

The second difference between donating a kidney and saving a drowning person, is that when a person is drowning, there is no time to think. The plight of another person is so present, urgent and compelling that it makes it impossible think before acting. In one's gut, he or she knows that jumping in the water is crazy and dangerous, but nevertheless, instinctively reacts because it the natural thing to do. However, with kidney donation, there exists a buffer of time. This is where one can step back and process the fears and risks involved, and conduct a thoughtful cost/benefit analysis. It is within this analytic process that one has the opportunity to think and possibly decide to not "jump in."

However, in my own experience, it was this second factor – the benefit of time - that actually served as the greatest help in bringing me closer to my decision. Since I took my time, I was able to advance through the process carefully and methodically over the course of a year. I invested time to read, research and explore every possible perspective. I knew that if I was, in fact, going to donate a kidney, it would be with the confidence that I had been thorough in my research and answered the dozens of questions I had pondered and compiled.

3. Where does the process start?

Most goals in life focus on the end result. Thus, all of one's energies are concentrated on achieving those specific results. Yet, with kidney donation, it is not about the end-result. Whether or not one ultimately donates a kidney is, dare I say, less important than the process itself. It is not about the answers one receives, but about the questions that are asked. For through the questions one wrestles with, an amazing personal transformation occurs.

Every kidney donor has a unique starting point. For most people, they receive a tap on the shoulder from friends or family, asking them to consider donating a kidney. While most people are understandably shocked by the question, it is important to recognize how painfully difficult it is for a patient to ask. For those who need a kidney, there is terrible guilt associated with the process of asking others to put themselves at risk and even consider kidney donation. Yet, since it is a matter of life and death, there is little choice - asking of others is a matter of survival. Thus, when someone works up the courage to ask, they should not be quickly dismissed, but rather commended for having the strength to come forward and ask the question.

While the ultimate question they are asking is whether or not you would donate a kidney, it is not the starting point for the conversation. The real question that should be asked, is whether or not one would consider being **tested**, and open to exploring the possibility of kidney donation. This is because there are hundreds of baby steps along the way of this journey. Furthermore, for many people, even if they are willing to donate, they may not be a suitable candidate or match for kidney donation.

In my situation, the starting point was different - as I did not receive such a tap on the shoulder - it was a gradual process that unfolded over the course of twelve months. However, I eventually realized that, in truth, my journey began many years before I ever thought about kidney donation. For it is in the early development of every child that seeds are planted, which, under the right conditions can blossom long into the future.

I was blessed to be raised in a home that was full of love, where acts of kindness were the norm. Perhaps as a child I may not have appreciated the impact of my parents, grandparents, community and teachers. Yet, there is no doubt that many wonderful people have had profoundly positive influences on my giving nature.

One such example became clear to me only two years ago when I was waiting in a checkout line at the store. I noticed a teenager standing ahead of me nervously counting a handful of change. The cashier added up the price of his items and said, "that will be ten dollars." The young man began to stammer as he realized he did not have enough money, and was trying to decide which of his purchases to return.

I leaned over to the cashier with a smile and told him to put the difference on my bill. The teenager turned around and looked at me with an expression on his face as if he had just won the lottery. He was so deeply touched by the simple gesture of a total stranger. Yet, in my own mind something else was happening. As he profusely thanked me, I was transformed back to my childhood to relive a memory that I had not thought about in nearly thirty years.

I recalled being in summer camp on a hot July day, as a boy of nine or ten years old. After spending weeks saving up loose change, I excitedly ran up to the top of the hill to purchase a cold can of soda from the camp's new soda machine. One after another I carefully inserted the coins. Reaching up to deposit the last dime, it accidentally slipped between my fingers, fell to the floor and rolled beneath the soda machine. I quickly dropped to the ground and tried sliding my little fingers under the machine to retrieve my dime. As hard as I tried, I was unable to reach it, and feeling devastated and defeated, I gave up.

As I turned away from the machine, I was greeted by the sight of a tall man approaching. He took one look at my face and asked what was wrong. I explained that I put my money in but dropped the last coin and could not reach it. Without hesitating, he smiled and reached into his pocket, pulling out a handful of change and helped me purchase my can of soda. I looked up at him and innocently asked, "how should I pay you back?"

He looked at me with a very serious expression and said, "this is how you should pay me back: when you are an adult, you are going to see another child trying to buy a can of soda who does not have enough money. I want you to go over to that child and give him the money he needs."

Thirty years had gone by without ever thinking about that story. Yet, in that very moment standing in the checkout line at the store, I instinctively reached out to offer the young man the money he needed. Such is the power of planting seeds of kindness in the hearts and minds of other people. It is this story and many others which, throughout my life, have collectively contributed to my willingness to explore ways to help other people.

In fact, I was raised watching my grandfather excuse himself on the weekends, so that he could walk several miles each way to go nursing homes, where he would visit total strangers. As he put it, he would sing and dance for the residents and flirt with the old ladies, knowing it would bring a big smile to their faces. I watched as he took the talents he was blessed with and used them to bring joy and hope to others. Observing his passion for kindness was a game-changer in my own young development. As a result, I have learned that one should never underestimate the impact every little act of kindness can have, not just on the recipient, but on the giver and the giver's entire family.

4. What exactly does a kidney do?

This may seem like an obvious question, but before I embarked upon my journey, I had to stop and ask. After all, I was blessed with two great kidneys my entire life, and since I had never experienced any problems, I did not really give thought to what they do. In my research, I learned that kidneys carry out numerous complicated and precise functions. They are involved in the regulation of systems which include electrolytes, pH levels, glucose, amino acids, hormones and enzymes. The kidneys essentially act as a state-of-the-art filter: they take in blood, purify it, and then produce urine to eliminate the waste and toxins.

When a person has poor kidney function, he or she is unable to filter out harmful impurities from the bloodstream, resulting in the body filling with deadly toxins, which could quickly lead to death. Essentially, having healthy kidneys means the difference between life and death.

5. What is dialysis?

Dialysis is a process during which a person's blood is drawn out, filtered of waste and toxins, and returned back to their body. This is also referred to as hemodialysis The medical advancements that exist today are remarkable. With dialysis, a person that does not have proper kidney function can be connected to a dialysis machine which acts as a mechanical kidney.

The problem is that even the best dialysis, the machine does only about 15% of what a healthy kidney can do and it is extremely time consuming. When a person is connected to dialysis, he or she spends at least 4 hours at a time, three days per week, being tethered to this machine, preventing them from maintaining the rhythm of a normal life.

Recently, select locations have begun offering nocturnal dialysis, which affords patients the opportunity to show up for an evening appointment in their pajamas, receive dialysis while they sleep, and return to work in the morning. This allows them to continue living life, while they wait for a new kidney. Yet, not every kidney patient is a suitable candidate to receive a transplant and dialysis becomes the key to survival and prolonging life.

Another form of dialysis is peritoneal dialysis, in which a catheter is surgically placed into the patient's stomach creating an artificial and temporary dialysis system that is maintained on a daily basis within the body of the patient. Although each form of dialysis has pros and cons, both are only temporary solutions.

6. Why can't a person just live on dialysis?

While some dialysis patients have lived as long as 20-30 years, the average person only survives 5-10 years on dialysis. During that time, the body continues to suffer and fight the toxin buildup. The good news is that some patients report feeling pretty good after dialysis. However, even in the best case scenario, for many people this only lasts for about one day. Within hours, the body begins to build up toxins again, leaving a person feeling fatigued, and making it difficult to return to their normal routine

The mental toll is as burdensome as the physical toll and sometimes greater. One dialysis patient explained to me that his mind actually suffered more than his body. He constantly felt as if he was in a haze and was unable to think clearly. He could not return to work, nor properly interact with his family.

Thus, dialysis is a wonderful way to temporarily prolong life. It is neither a cure, nor a solution to having failed or diseased kidneys, rather, it is a temporary bandage. People generally stop dialysis for two reasons: either they receive a much-needed kidney transplant, or, sadly, due to death.

7. How long can a patient wait for a kidney?

Unfortunately, once a patient is put on the transplant list, there is a long road toward receiving a kidney. This waiting game will last anywhere from 3-9 years, based upon what state a person lives in. Research has shown that, while some people can live as long as 20 years, 90% will die within 10 years of being on dialysis waiting for a kidney. **The average**

person on dialysis only lives for 5-6 years. Recent studies have shown that on average, 12 people in the United States die each day while waiting for a kidney donation.

8. How many people are waiting for a kidney transplant?

As of this writing, there are more than 100,000 people in the United States alone that are awaiting a life-saving kidney transplant, and over 4 million people worldwide. Kidney patients are regular people spanning all ages, races, and religions, and they live each day with the pressures of a ticking time-bomb, anxiously awaiting that phone call, informing them a donor kidney has been found.

Considering there are more than 320 million people in the United States, if only a fraction of 1% of Americans considered kidney donation, the entire list of 100,000 could quickly be reduced to zero.

When I first looked at the daunting number of 100,000, I remember skeptically telling myself, that even if I made the decision to donate a kidney, I would be risking my own life for the chance to lower that huge number by just one. It does not even make a dent and it hardly seems worth the risk. However, I soon

realized that it was not only about one person –
because to their children, siblings, parents and friends,
this was not about a number. Through the
preservation of a single life, it would create ripples that
would exponentially impact many lives.

That one number represents a daughter whose
father can walk her down the aisle at her wedding; or
a grandmother that can watch her grandchildren grow
up; or a child that lives a normal and healthy life.
Saving a life is not only about reducing that large
number by one, but it is about changing the lives of
countless people around the "one."

There is an ancient Talmudic dictum which states
that saving a single life is tantamount to saving the
entire world. This perspective suggests that an
individual is not a number, but a world unto
themselves and everyone around them. Thus, my
perspective began to shift when I asked myself how
far I would I be willing to go to save the entire world.

9.   Why do I have two kidneys if I only need one?

Throughout my research I was surprised to learn
that a person can live a perfectly normal life with only
one kidney. In fact, 1 out of every 750 people is

actually born with only one kidney. This condition is known as Unilateral Renal Agenesis, and most people born with one kidney never even realize it and live a normal and healthy life.

Medically speaking, the benefit of two kidneys is that if one is injured, the other can compensate. Therefore, as you will read later, if a person donates a kidney, he or she is relying that much more on the remaining kidney and must be mindful as they go through life to not take extra risks which could endanger their remaining kidney.

The more I pondered the question of why I was blessed with two kidneys if I only needed one, the more I realized how simple the answer was. It was so I would have the option of giving it to someone else who needed it. While it may seem like an overly-simplistic answer, I often hear the same response from countless kidney donors. We do not view it as our second kidney, but rather, as our extra kidney.

10. Isn't the second kidney a good backup just in case one gets damaged?

Having two kidneys can definitely be a great backup in the event that something happens to one of them. For instance, if a person playing tackle football suffers bodily injury and one kidney is damaged, the other will be able to compensate. In fact, there have been many people who have injured a kidney, but never knew about it, as their other kidney continued to do the work for both of them.

However, the majority of kidney-related problems which require a transplant, actually stem from illness. Thus, with regard to kidney disease, having two kidneys does not necessarily protect a person more than if he or she only had one. When kidney disease strikes, typically both kidneys get damaged simultaneously. Therefore, although a person might have two kidneys, when he or she is afflicted with this terrible illness, dialysis and transplant are the likely outcome.

11. How exactly does kidney donation work?

There are two forms of living-kidney donation. The first is a direct or targeted donation, where someone donates to a person they know. This is the most common form, such as in the case where a donation is made to a friend or family member.

The second is known as a non-directed donation, where a person donates to a total stranger. This is commonly referred to as an *altruistic donation*, although all donations are deeply altruistic. In both cases, one of the kidneys is taken from the donor and transplanted into the abdomen of the recipient. Following the transplant, the donor's remaining kidney enlarges and does the work of both kidneys, and for the recipient, the new kidney does the same. The transplant removes the need for dialysis, and allows the recipient to begin living a normal life.

12. How common is altruistic donation?

Unfortunately, even with over 100,000 people in the United States awaiting a kidney donation, the waiting list continues to get longer and longer. Intuitively, one might suspect that as medical advancements continue to develop, the number of people on the waiting list would decrease. However, the opposite has happened. Doctors have found ways to prolong life for patients on dialysis, ultimately buying them more time as they wait for a donation. Yet, our society has not significantly increased the number of donations to match the growing demand.

Sadly, there are very few altruistic kidney donations taking place each year. In 2014 the UK reported only 100 such donations, and in the United States, only several hundred altruistic donations - where good Samaritans have donated to total strangers

- have taken place. This is the statistic which I believe can change with increased awareness and many more lives can be saved through the largesse of total strangers.

13. Can't you just use a kidney from a cadaver?

Before I made any decisions about donating a vital organ, I had to understand why doctors were taking organs from living patients, instead of cadavers, (also known as deceased donation). In my research, I learned that cadaveric or deceased kidney transplants happen all the time and are highly successful. If that were the case, it made no sense for me to put myself at risk to donate my kidney.

However, there are a number of issues with a kidney from a cadaver. The first issue is the limited availability. As an example, in the event that a person was in a tragic motor vehicle accident and declared brain-dead, the doctor's must determine if that person (or their family by proxy) agreed to organ donation. Next, they must ascertain whether the organs are healthy and viable for transplantation. Finally, if the answer was yes to both questions, a match must be quickly found. Once the kidney is harvested from the cadaver, it has very little time to be implanted. The longer it remains outside of the body, the more compromised the organ will be. Even if the transplant were to be done quickly enough, the kidney, which was previously dead, must then be resuscitated. In many cases, it works right away. However, often, the kidney takes days, weeks or months to achieve its full level of functioning, and sometimes it does not even work at all. In these cases, the patient with the transplanted kidney may remain in the hospital for extended periods of time, increasing the risks of further complications. In the event that the transplanted kidney fails, the patient who recently underwent surgery and is in the process of recovering, must once again begin dialysis and be put back on the list, as they wait all over again for an additional transplant.

Moreover, research has shown that on average, a deceased-donor kidney tends not to last as long, in comparison to a kidney donated by a living donor. These conditions make it possible, but less than ideal to use a deceased donor's kidney, if a living donor's kidney is available.

There is no doubt that when people sign the back of their driver's license and agree to donate their organs, they are making a remarkable commitment to save lives. However, the reality is only 1% of people die in a way that allows their organs to be used. Nevertheless, while that number is low, imagine how many countless lives can be saved if just 1% of our population took that pledge and expressed their commitment to sharing organs to save lives!

14. How long does a kidney last?

Amazingly, the kidneys we were born with can last a lifetime and even beyond! That's right. There are stories of people who have donated a kidney later in life, and decades later when the donor passed away, their kidney continued to function within the recipient long beyond the rest of the donor's body! The way I see it, even though the donor may be gone, he or she continues to live on through their recipient.

A donated kidney can last anywhere from a few years to a number of decades. On average 50% of donated kidneys last 18-20 years. Remember, most people keep their own functioning kidneys for their entire lives; they were built to last! However, in someone else's body, the kidney faces the challenge of having to survive in a potentially hostile environment that cannot tell if the new kidney belongs there, or if it should be attacked as a foreign body and threat.

There are many factors that will contribute to the health and longevity of the donated kidney, including how well the recipient takes care of his or her own health. Additionally, if the cross-matching is a close fit, the kidney may even last longer, and less long-term anti-rejection medications would be required. Furthermore, as medical advancements continue, there are constant improvements to the quality of the post-transplant medications, which further allow the kidney to live a long and healthy life.

When I began this process, I assumed that donating a kidney meant that it would remain with the recipient for the rest of their lives. I have to admit, that when I first learned that donated kidneys will not necessarily last forever, I was somewhat disappointed and discouraged. I did not feel up to going through all of this, just to imagine that the kidney might fail in five, ten or twenty years. Then, I really spent time reflecting on this one point.

While the health and diet of the recipient can impact the kidney's longevity, ultimately, I realized that it was out of my control. Perhaps a donated kidney will last ten years, maybe it will last thirty. I started to question whether that unknown detail should be a deterrent for me. One fact which I clearly knew was that dialysis is ultimately a slow-death sentence, during which a patient will almost certainly deteriorate and die over the next decade. I realized that if I could extend a person's life by even ten years (with the possibility of twenty or thirty), is that not of great value? Would I not wish for someone to do the same for me? How could I minimize what ten years means to a mother who is watching her children grow up, or a grandfather being alive to dance with his granddaughter at her wedding?

I came to the conclusion, that giving someone even an extra five, ten or twenty years is very much the definition of saving a life. Furthermore, by extending someone's life for that amount of time, it does not mean that their life will then end. Instead, I am giving them the opportunity to make it to the next chapter in their lives. Perhaps in twenty years medical technology will be far improved, or synthetic kidneys (which are already being researched and developed) will be available to take them the rest of the way.

It took me some time and a lot of soul searching, but I eventually came to realize what an important role I would be playing in extending someone's life, even if it were on a limited basis, and helping a person who is on dialysis return to a normal and wonderful life. When I look at how the life of my own recipient has been improved just over the last several years, I am amazed and awed by the opportunity she was given to start an entirely new life. Ronit has watched her children continue to grow up, graduate high school and get married. Ronit has even successfully put herself through law school and started a new career as an attorney!

Is any human being qualified to determine whether five, ten or twenty years is considered valuable?

According to my own value system, I view every moment of life as being sacred. Thus, when I look at the endless joys and accomplishments of Ronit just over the last few short years, I am completely amazed, gratified and humbled by how meaningfully she embraces each moment of each and every day!

Chapter 2:
The Testing Process

15. What is the very first step in exploring the kidney donation process?

This is the first step -by researching and reading a book like this, one is able to become educated, so he or she can make an informed decision. Keep in mind, donating a kidney is not a decision made at the beginning of the process! Rather, the actual decision comes at the end. There are about a dozen important steps in the process along the way, and no commitment is truly made, until the surgery actually begins. It is important for potential donors to be aware that they have the right and the ability to walk away at any point prior to the surgery.

Being informed and educated is an important part of the process. Keep in mind that the Internet is a wonderful resource that will provide countless amazing kidney donation stories, as well as negative donation experiences. I found it helpful to read them all. In fact, the more I read, the more I understood about the process and knew what questions to ask.

In all honesty, by reading some of the negative, or more sobering accounts of kidney donation, I was quickly turned off. On numerous occasions, I would exit my browser, shut the computer and walk away from the entire concept, only to return weeks later after having had time to properly process these stories.

I soon realized the negative stories were often the exceptions and not the norm. Just like anything in life, there will always be people who have bad experiences. Whether booking a hotel, buying electronics or a new car, choosing a doctor or lawyer, we have access today to read countless reviews of the experiences of other people. Even when almost everyone reports a positive experience, it does not guarantee that there won't be exceptions. Every five-star review will also be balanced by a one-star experience. The difference between an online purchase and kidney donation however, is that negative experiences with kidney donation can mean a catastrophic outcome for one's health or life. For me, as frightening and real as those stories were, I wanted to hear them as well, so that I would not go through this process blindly or naively. I needed to understand the range of possible risks, including physical, emotional or financial ramifications, and of course, death.

While kidney donation is certainly a beautiful and meaningful experience, it was important for me to not go into it wearing rose-colored glasses. I felt that the more information I had to make my decision, the better off I would be.

16. Who can be a kidney donor?

Like many people, I was under a false impression that finding a suitable kidney donor was a near impossible task. For years, I have heard about people asking for bone marrow donors to come forward. These campaigns attempted to attract the maximum number of people to be tested and entered into a registry in the hopes of finding a rare, but suitable match. This is because finding a donor for a bone marrow transplant is tantamount to finding a needle in a haystack.

When it came to kidneys, I assumed that donation was so rare because the same must be true. However, I soon learned that the reality is that most adults of average to good health could be considered potential candidates for kidney donation. Unlike bone marrow donors, to donate a kidney one is not required to have special DNA matching.

Understanding this helped me appreciate that kidney donation is particularly accessible. The low number of donations were not a result of struggling to find the single person with the right strand of DNA, rather, the challenge was simply to find anyone with a healthy kidney who was willing to part with it.

17. How do I know if I am a match?

To be a match, the basic criterion is that you must be the same blood type as the recipient. Someone with an A blood type (regardless of negative or positive) can donate to another person with an A blood type. The same is true for someone whose B blood type is B, they can donate to another B blood type. Anyone with a blood type of O is considered a universal donor that can donate to anyone.

Therefore, if a person is donating to someone specific, such as a friend or family member, the first step is to know what the recipient's blood type is. However, since there can be numerous factors involved, knowing the blood type alone does not guarantee that one is a fully compatible donor. That is where the testing phase can help provide more information.

In my case, I was not looking to donate to anyone specific. I simply felt that I was blessed with the gift of an extra kidney, which I was not specifically using, and was happy to give to someone else who needed it more than I did. Therefore, as an A+ blood type, I knew that if I would donate, it would be to a recipient who also had an A blood type.

18. What is cross-matching?

After matching blood type, the donor is tested against a specific recipient to determine that their cross-matching is negative.

This is where the cells of the donors and recipient are combined in a lab to observe how they react. Either they will coexist, indicating that the match is suitable, or the antibodies of the recipient will begin attacking the cells of the donor, which suggests that the two are incompatible. There can also be a wide range of degree to which the cells of the donor and recipient struggle to coexist. The more closely the two are matched, the more likely the recipient's body will accept the kidney without much of a fight.

As a general rule, anyone that receives a transplant, will take anti-rejection medication for the rest of their lives. These medications help suppress the recipient's immunity, so their own body does not attack the kidney as a foreign object in their body. The better the cross-matching is between the donor and recipient, the more likely the kidney will thrive in its new body with less anti-rejection medication required.

What is important to remember is that a donor's HLA (which helps measure the antigens and compatibility) does not need to be a perfect match to a recipient, but the closer the better. Moreover, with ongoing progress in this medical arena, new breakthroughs for improving compatibility are constantly being researched and discovered.

19. Why do some people talk about compensation for kidney donation?

It is critical to realize early on that for many people who are walking the line between life and death, they are desperate to do anything to live, including pay high sums of money. At the same time, there are people living in abject poverty, who would do most anything to feed and support their families. As a result, there are "black-market" avenues for kidney exchange that one should be aware of, and avoid on all accounts. It is both illegal and unethical for a person to pay or receive money for donating a kidney.

Consider the fact that when people are acting illegally or going underground to trade organs for money, they are not only violating ethical principles, but putting countless people at risk by compromising the medical quality and the numerous safety nets our system puts in place to protect both the donors and recipients. In situations where people travel to other countries and engage in buying and selling of organs, the rates of long-term health problems and death increase dramatically. I have read many stories of people who have taken this route, received a large sum of money in exchange for a kidney, and then spent the rest of their lives in and out of hospitals trying to recover from health-problems associated with a careless surgical procedure.

A kidney donation should never include any form of compensation, no matter how lucrative the offer may be. The only form of financial compensation that is legally and ethically permitted is reimbursement for the donor's expenses associated with the donation. These may include travel costs, child and home care during the recovery process, and even lost-wages.

20. Who should I talk to in order to learn more?

There are a number of local and national non-profit kidney organizations that are dedicated to helping altruistic kidney donors walk through the process of exploring whether kidney donation is right for them. Most transplant centers and major hospitals will also offer such services. Often, hospitals are staffed by a transplant coordinator whose job it is to speak with potential donors and provide the education, resources, and information that will help them to become most informed. One can easily search online to explore the many resources and options, ranging from transplant hospitals to non-profit organizations and faith-based agencies that exist in their own community, as well as nationally and globally. One should not be afraid to speak to people from these agencies, as they live each day waiting to speak to ordinary people who are simply interested in learning more about kidney donation.

21. Why is it so hard for me to pick up the phone and inquire about kidney donation?

For months I agonized over picking up the phone. I had spent hundreds of hours researching and thinking about kidney donation, and I still did not even know if I was a suitable match, or in proper health to donate. Yet, I could not bring myself to pick up the phone and make that first call.

While I knew in my heart that I had made no commitment, a part of me was very nervous, as if by making this first phone call, I was somewhat bound. It would be as if I had formally started the process and was now officially in the system, though I was nowhere ready to begin the process. All I wanted to do was speak to someone who could offer further guidance. This was a struggle that raged within me for months.

Looking back, I believe that this inner turmoil was a very healthy struggle. It meant that I did not rush into my decision, and instead, was going about it in a cautious and thoughtful manner.

However, I wish that at the time, instead of agonizing about whether or not to call, someone would have just put an arm around me and explained that making that call was not about making any commitments. It was actually the best way to alleviate my stress and uncertainty by allowing me to speak with other people who better understood the process and could explain it to me clearly. Making that first phone call would give me the space to discuss my concerns and stop needlessly worrying about so many theoretical variables.

For me, part of the challenge in making that first phone call was that I had so thoroughly researched kidney donation, I was not really calling to learn about the topic - I already knew much of the facts, the risks involved, and even the benefits. What I really needed to figure out what was I would say when I picked up the phone. Eventually, I came to realize that making that first phone call was about learning how kidney donation related to me personally.

Perhaps that was the part that frightened me the most. At that early stage, I did not even know my blood type or whether I would be a good candidate. Perhaps I was agonizing for nothing and would be told based on my family's medical history that I was not even a good candidate. Or, alternatively, I was concerned that someone would tell me, "you sound great, come on in, we can get you in for surgery next Tuesday." I was simply unsure what to expect. I feared that by making that phone call, it would all become very real, very quickly.

As it turned out, I could not have been more wrong. Picking up the phone and finally calling was the most empowering step in helping me learn that the process was actually far less rushed than I expected.

While this first phone call is an important step, potential donors should not allow themselves to get discouraged if they call and have a difficult time reaching someone. The reality is, transplant coordinators are often quite swamped as they work so passionately to help save lives, juggling and coordinating dozens of cases on any given day.

Additionally, some donors have found the person on the other end of the phone sounding somewhat distant, rather than eager and excited to speak with them. It is important to recognize that this is not because the coordinator lacks personality, but rather, he or she may deliberately come across as even-keeled, so their tone not be misinterpreted as coercive. Because of the sensitive nature and ethical considerations of kidney donation, hospitals and transplant centers try to walk a fine line of being fully supportive and encouraging of donors, without being pushy. Therefore, if at first one does not get the answers or information that he or she is looking for, remember the careful balancing act that the hospital is playing, and try again.

22. What should I expect on the first phone call?

After months of research, I finally found the courage to make that first phone call to a non-profit kidney agency, which I had read about in a community magazine. My conversation was surprisingly far more pleasant than I anticipated. I was offered brochures and information, and given a general roadmap outlining the overall process. This included the many steps between inquiring and testing, all the way through the donation and recovery. I was asked a few questions about my general health, and was invited to ask anything that was on my mind. When I hung up from that first forty-five-minute phone call, I felt far more at ease than I did before. I now felt I knew someone specific I could talk to (who happened to also be a kidney donor herself).

Although I still had many questions to ask, and a great deal of information to still learn, my primary question at this stage was whether or not I was wasting my time. After all, my family history of heart disease and high blood pressure was not very promising. In fact, I was fairly convinced that I would be disqualified as a candidate and would then be allowed to resume my life as normal, with a good feeling on my conscience for having tried to do a good deed.

In order to gain clarity and know whether to cross this idea off my list, or to continue pursuing it, I needed to understand whether I was even a viable candidate. This process required a close look at my health and medical history. So, after receiving a recommendation, I contacted Pat, the Transplant Coordinator at Montefiore Medical Center in New York. She, too, put me at ease by simply addressing my many questions. At the end of the call, she asked, "how would you feel if I emailed you some paperwork so that you can fill out your medical history, which will then give us a general idea about your candidacy, and then we can go from there?"

I really appreciated that as a next step. Paperwork? I can handle paperwork. It was simple, practical and completely non-invasive! In fact, I felt as if that step was really able to help me progress. After all, I was growing more curious whether or not I could even be a donor. By filling out the medical forms, it allowed me to simply take that next step in exploration of how kidney donation related to me, albeit, without making any commitment. Additionally, as I looked through the paperwork, reading through the extensive list of disorders, diseases and illnesses, I realized just how many items I was blessed to be able to check that little box that read "no." This really helped me count my blessings and gain perspective as to why I felt so compelled to continue to explore this process.

I reflected on the endless number of things that could go wrong with a person's health, and for some unknown reason, I was blessed to be free from most all of them. With that heightened sense of appreciation for the many blessings in my life, I felt more confident about using what I was given to help others in need.

23. Can I still be a donor if I have a complicated medical history?

The initial questionnaire includes basic biographical information and medical history. It is designed to give the medical team an overall snapshot of the donor's general health. They are clearly looking for family history of illnesses such as cancer, diabetes or kidney problems. But here is the surprising part, just because one might have had a bumpy medical history, does not mean that he or she would not be a good candidate for kidney donation.

I was fairly confident that with high blood pressure and heart disease in my family, I would not be a accepted as a candidate. Yet, I was shocked to learn that my concerns were not necessarily problematic for kidney donation, as the doctors do not look at each issue independently, but they look at the entire picture of one's health - past, present and future. The important take-away to remember from this part of the process is that one should not self-disqualify without first getting a professional opinion.

24. Who pays for all the testing?

The donor does not pay for any part of the evaluation process - either the recipient's insurance covers all of the costs for the testing, or the transplant center itself will cover the costs. This means, that a potential donor would receive the Cadillac of medical testing - what the doctors often refer to as the "million-dollar workup," at no cost to them. I actually welcomed this part of the process. Over the years, I have heard numerous stories of people that have gone to the doctor for a minor issue, and miraculously, the doctors discovered something major, which would have been life-threatening if undiagnosed. Only because it was accidentally discovered was the person's life ultimately saved. So too, I looked at the testing as an amazing opportunity that would yield one of three possibilities:

Option 1: I would be disqualified from kidney donation because of some obscure finding or family history and I could go about my life, feeling good for having tried to donate.

Option 2: I would be approved for kidney donation, verify that I was in perfect health, and then decide if it was something I wanted to do.

Option 3: I would learn that there was something else wrong with my health, which I never would have otherwise known about. Only through this series of testing, would my own life be saved.

As I weighed these three possible options, I realized that I was truly comfortable with any of the outcomes and decided to proceed with the testing process.

25. What kind of medical testing is required?

After submitting my paperwork, I was contacted one week later by the transplant coordinator. I was quite surprised when she told me that on paper I looked like a good candidate. She went on to explain that without actually doing a number of tests, there was no way to know for sure.

She asked if I was interested in exploring this further, explaining that the testing would allow the doctors to take a closer look at my body and health, and determine if kidney donation was even an option for me. Remember, at this point, I was still not committed, nor had I made a decision whether this was something I wanted to do. The testing stage was all about seeing if I was even a candidate, so that I could know whether or not there was a decision to be made in the future.

After she informed me that the initial testing simply included a urine and blood test, I gladly agreed to continue with the process.

Although the blood test was the same as any other I had ever received, they drew a number of extra tubes of blood, in order to thoroughly conduct the required tests. In all honesty, it was quick and rather painless. This step allowed doctors to confirm my blood type, check the health of my blood and look at my antigens and cross-matching.

The next step involved filling a cup for a urine-analysis. This allowed the doctors to evaluate my creatinine and protein levels, telling of the health and functioning of my kidneys. All of this basic information helps paint a preliminary picture as to whether or not, the donor seems suitable.

Following the urine and blood tests, I was surprised to get a call one week later, informing that my initial tests looked great. I was asked if I wanted to continue the testing to further explore my candidacy, without making any commitments whatsoever.

I was somewhat skeptical to proceed without knowing exactly what was involved. It was at this point that I was first introduced to the term "the million-dollar workup." This is where the doctors perform a series of very expensive tests (at no cost to the donor), to look at every aspect of his or her health. Not only were they looking for any problems with the kidney itself, but they examine if there is an increased likelihood of any systemic, cardiac, pulmonary, or renal issues developing in the future. The theme of looking out for the best interests of the donor emerged repeatedly throughout the process.

I agreed to have this thorough evaluation, and scheduled the next round of explorations. During this stage, an EKG was administered to look at my heart and a chest x-ray was taken to determine the health of my lungs. A CAT scan with contrast dye was performed to look more closely in my abdomen and determine the health of my organs and blood vessels. Finally, an ultrasound was done to get a closer look at my kidneys and the arteries which support their blood flow. The length of the renal arteries were a particular focus, to ensure they were long enough to properly connect the kidney to the recipient.

One of the most moving parts of the testing phase was sitting in the waiting room with renal patients and noticing the looks on their faces. There was a pervasive sadness permeating the environment. On numerous occasions I stuck up a conversation with others in the waiting room. Inevitably, when I mentioned I was being tested for donation, their faces would light up. It is hard to describe the look of hope reflected in their smiles, when they heard about one more life that might be saved.

I found that connecting with the patients, and appreciating what life was like for them, really helped me understand what this process was about. It was for that reason, that I welcomed the final test of this phase, which began with the nurse handing me a large plastic container and asked me to do a 24-hour urine collection (i.e. I would only urinate into the container for a 24-hour period). Initially, I was caught off guard by the request and my mind began racing to try and figure out the logistics of how exactly to make it work.

The nurse explained that it was important to assess the level of kidney function, and to measure how much urine they produced in an average 24-hour window, while measuring their creatinine and protein levels. I decided to find a convenient time over the weekend to perform the test, and made sure to never stray too far from the container!

More than any of the other tests, this one truly gave me a deeper connection to dialysis patients. Even though my test only lasted for 24 hours, it forced me to stop and consider what life must be like for many of the kidney patients who cannot simply use the restroom at their convenience. It gave me pause and helped me further appreciate how blessed I was to have two perfectly healthy kidneys.

Overall, in my experience, I found the testing to be extremely smooth and easy. I was only further amazed, when the hospital's transplant coordinator came running after me as I was heading out from an afternoon of tests and appointments. I was caught off guard and asked what was wrong, or if there was something I missed. She smiled saying, "no, not at all, I just wanted to validate your parking, so that you do not incur any expenses during this process."

26. Can I choose to whom I will donate?

Yes. A donor has the full right to direct or approve to whom they are giving their kidney and should never feel pressure to donate to someone specific. Most living kidney donations today are targeted or directed donations, which means they are giving to a specific person, such as a friend or family member. Thus, they work together with their local hospital to conduct the testing and ultimately, the transplant to the intended recipient.

For me, while I was open to donating to anyone, I saw kidney donation as an opportunity to give back to those around me. Therefore, I drew concentric circles to try and identify if I knew of someone in need. I started by looking to see if anyone in my family may have been in need of a kidney. When that search turned up empty, I continued to expand my circles to look within my faith-community, as if I were donating to a member of my extended family. It was this exploration which led me to discover that within many faith-based communities, there are grass-root support groups and agencies that will help dialysis patients to find matches. I found a number of such non-profit organizations in my own Jewish community that were able to help provide me with the information and direction that I needed.

27. How do I get matched?

Each transplant hospital coordinates with UNOS (United Network for Organ Sharing) and maintains lists and databases of patients who are eligible for a transplant, as well as prospective donors. If a donor comes forward with a specific person to whom they wish to donate to, the transplant coordinator will work directly to explore the feasibility of the match.

However, for donors who do not have a particular recipient in mind, it can be a very different experience. Remember, there is no obligation to donate to anyone the hospital recommends as a good match. For example, if the hospital suggests that they have a worthy match who is a 76 years old patient, one may decide that he or she would rather donate to save the life of a child. Since every single life is precious, no matter how old or young, this is a very difficult decision to make, and many people undergo some stress and guilt in trying to decide. One may even feel uncomfortable, as if they are playing God, deciding who should live and who should die.

Nevertheless, since the organ is the donor's to give, donors have the full right to think about what type of recipient speaks to them. Even if the choice does not seem fully "rational," it is the donor's right to make the decision without any pressure. Because of the complexity of making this choice, some would prefer not to deal with this aspect, and instead, simply instruct the transplant coordinator to pair them with the next suitable match on the list, whoever it may be.

28. If I am not a match to someone specific, can I still donate?

There is an option which is known as the paired-exchange, or the "domino donation." This happens when a person is willing to give a kidney to save the life of a friend or family member, but unfortunately, he or she is not a match to their intended recipient. However, they match an unrelated person who has the exact same dilemma, causing a chain reaction or domino effect.

For instance, A wishes to donate to B, but is not a match. In another city or state, C wishes to donate to D but is not a match. What the hospital can research and coordinate, is to mix and match these two families, so that A can donate to D, and C to B. It takes some maneuvering and coordination between the sets of donors and recipients, but in these cases, while each donor is giving a kidney to a stranger, each recipient gets a healthy kidney. By doing this type of a swap, it is a win-win for both recipients in need. In fact, some donors prefer to find a paired-exchange, so that their single donation not only helps save the life of one recipient, but can actually save the lives of a number of people who are in need of a kidney!

If perhaps this sounds complicated trying to coordinate between two families, imagine when there are five or even ten families, who are all lined up to donate to the next one. This domino-like strategy takes a great deal of work and planning, but with access to larger databases, these types of donations are becoming more and more common.

29. How do they choose which of my two kidneys to take?

Typically, the donor's left kidney is selected for donation, as it is more easily transplanted due to the lengthier blood vessels, making it easier to attach to the recipient. Additionally, statistics have demonstrated that in the event of bodily injury (such as a car accident), the left kidney is more susceptible to harm. Therefore, by transplanting the left kidney, it increases the likelihood that the remaining right kidney will be safe and protected. Not only are extra measures constantly taken to look out for the best interest of the recipient, but to also ensure that the donor's remaining kidney will be as safely protected as possible.

However, for a variety of medical reasons, doctors may explore either kidney for donation. Each case is assessed individually and the doctors will determine which kidney is better fit for transplant. The primary factor in choosing which kidney to transplant will always be determined upon the medical advantages of the kidney and protecting the health of the donor.

30. Who pays for the surgery?

This was a significant concern as I began the journey. I was reassured that all of the medical tests leading up to the surgery were covered by the recipient's insurance, however, I wanted to know specifically about the surgery itself. Even though I had medical insurance which covered surgeries, I was concerned that since this was an elective procedure, it may not be covered. Furthermore, even if it were covered by my insurance, an expensive surgery could potentially leave me with the high costs of copays and deductibles.

Therefore, I was relieved to learn that all of the medical costs associated with the surgery including the costs for the medical testing and the relevant follow-up care after the surgery are covered by the recipient's insurance. However, it does not cover the donor's long-term healthcare. For instance, if a donor experiences complications, and as a result lives with ongoing donation-related problems, he or she should not expect the transplant center to cover the lifelong healthcare costs. Instead, it is important for donors to have their own insurance to care for themselves following the initial recovery process. In fact, there are numerous transplant centers that will not accept donors who do not have health insurance. This is not an act of discrimination against people without insurance. On the contrary, it is to protect them. Even though hospitals want to encourage more transplants, they do not wish to accept donors that may be left in a compromised or vulnerable health situation without the means of getting the medical help they may need in the future.

31. Am I responsible to pay for any extra expenses that come up along the way?

Although all medical expenses are covered, there may still be additional costs which arise, which are not necessarily covered by insurance. For instance, a donor may wish to take a taxi home from the hospital, or hire babysitting help for one's children during the recuperation. While these are expenses due to the kidney donation, as they are not direct medical expenses, one should investigate to see if they will be covered by insurance.

There are other avenues one can explore, that may provide reimbursements for a variety of donor-related expenses. This can best be accomplished by working with an agency, foundation, charity, or non-profit organization that may help cover additional costs. While these funds are not endless, they are specifically allocated to help encourage people to consider kidney donation, without having any financial burdens. I have also seen people successfully launch online crowd-funding campaigns, where they are able to have family, friends and even total strangers make contributions to help offset any added expenses.

Personally, I was fortunate to work with a faith-based organization that helped cover any added costs or expenses associated with the kidney donation – I did not even need to spend one penny out of pocket. Remember, while one may never receive any form of payment for donating a kidney, it does not mean that one should lose money either. When donation-related costs arise, such as lost wages; transportation to and from the hospital or appointments; or even domestic help at home while one recovers, these donation-related costs may be covered by doing one's research, and speaking with a variety of agencies dedicated to supporting donors.

32. What are the risks of dying?

This is THE big question and it should not be taken lightly. After all, kidney donation is a major surgery and as with all major surgeries, there is a risk of death. Personally, I live with the belief that when my time has come and my number is called, that is when my life is over. That does not mean I should take extreme risks and tempt fate. Rather, I am compelled to live life fully, yet responsibly. Within my own belief system, I feel there are certain ideals that are greater than myself. Thus, living life to the fullest truly means pushing it to the limit and finding the greatest purpose in one's existence.

Every day, firefighters and police officers risk their lives for a purpose greater than themselves. Their existential pursuit allows them to risk life and limb to save the lives of other people. It is a noble calling that does not come without danger. However, with proper preparation and training their odds of survival increase and it becomes a risk they are willing to take.

The general medical literature suggests that the mortality rate for living kidney donation is .03%. This means that 3 out of 10,000 people die from the surgery. However, some research studies report statistics which reflect a slightly higher number of 4 out of 10,000. It is recommended to check with each specific transplant center and ask what their particular statistics are, for some may report worse outcomes and many will report far better than the national average.

The biggest problem I had when I heard the number "0.03%" is that it is just a number. It did not really resonate with me or give me a good sense of what it really means. Do I even know 10,000 people? Could my mind truly grasp what losing 3 in 10,000 actually means? Are those good odds or bad odds?

Did you know?

- 1 in 3000 people will be struck by lightning at some point during their lifetime.

- 1 in 4,238 people die each year from falling out of a bed or chair.

- 1 in 5000 people will die in an automobile accident.

If I would simply rely on statistics to make my decision, I could argue that more people die each year from bicycle accidents than from kidney donations. Does that mean that kidney donation is without risk, or that I should stop riding my bike? Certainly not. Everything we do in life comes with risk.

The problem with trying to make a decision based solely on statistics, is that for the one person who actually dies in each statistic – the numbers are simply irrelevant. For them, the statistic is 100%. It means their life is over, regardless of the odds. We all want to be risk-averse to the extent that we can still live life to the fullest. To remain in bed every day for fear of death or injury, might be a way to stay alive, but by my definition, it is not living.

As I continued to research kidney donation, I spent months pondering these statistics to try and make sense of them. Every day, people undergo surgery, whether to have a hip or knee replaced, a tummy-tuck or facelift, or to have an appendix or gallbladder removed. Each of these "routine" surgeries come with the risk of general anesthesia and have their own mortality statistics and risk factors. Nevertheless, I realized that most people do not view these surgeries as a frightening and risky brush with death, rather, a daily part of life that must be confronted and overcome.

When a woman conceives a child, she spends nine months allowing her body to be overrun by her developing child – likely without giving thought to her mortality. She willingly endures the risks and excruciating pains of labor and childbirth - and for what? To give life to another human being! As I pondered this, I wondered why it is socially acceptable for women to risk their lives to have children, but donating a kidney – which is also life giving - was considered so outrageous?

According to the World Health Organization, in 2014 the maternal mortality rate in the United States was 28 deaths per 100,000. More simply put, 2.8 women out of every 10,000 will die in childbirth. Compare this statistic with the kidney donation mortality rate, which is 3 out of 10,000 - and the numbers are almost identical.

Yet, have you ever met a woman (provided she is in good health) who chooses to not have children based upon the risk? Do couples harp on these statistics before starting a family? Of course not. They accept that when it comes to something as incredible as giving life - even though there may be risk involved - they are risks worth taking!

Simply put, life is so incredibly precious and sacred, it motivates people to go to great lengths. While, as a man, I may never experience the beauties of childbirth, through kidney donation, I got a glimpse of what it means to go out on a ledge and wholly give of oneself and their body to give the gift of life to another person – a risk unquestionably worth taking.

Chapter 3.
Weighing The Risks
& Making a Decision

33. How do I begin to make such an important decision?

Making this weighty decision begins like any other important decision – with information gathering. Whether a person is in the market to buy a new car; piece of technology; or a home, today's world of information allows one to thoroughly research and explore before making a purchase. During this process, it is important to keep in mind that information and opinion will run the full spectrum, because no matter how high-end a purchase may be, there will always be reports of those who have had a bad experience. It is almost unheard of to find the perfect 5-start rating without some complaints. Embracing this caveat, and in an effort to be fully informed, I continued to scour the Internet with an open mind, searching for both the positive and negative stories of kidney donors.

I remember the feelings of inspiration as I read about the many success stories. I also recall the feelings of dread and fear as I came across someone's account of a negative experience. Whether it was someone who suffered complications, such as developing an infection or fever; living with chronic pain; or just slow to recover, I began to realize and absorb the permanence of this decision. On a number of occasions, I even closed my laptop and walked away, not able to revisit the topic for weeks. I found that reading negative reports was discouraging, but at the same time, I continued to look for them, so that when I made my final decision, it would be based upon <u>all</u> points of view. I was not about to be naive regarding such an important decision. It took me weeks or months to process and reconcile the stories of those who had negative experiences. Over time, it became very clear that the negative stories were the exceptions and not the rule. In almost all cases, kidney donors were glad with the decision they made, and would do it again if they could.

While the Internet provided me with a great deal of information - both positive and negative, I learned to appreciate each point within the context it was given. For instance, much of the information I received came from message boards which were five or ten years old, which in the world of cutting-edge medical technology can be a lifetime. Furthermore, upon probing more deeply I realized that some, but not all, of the negative experiences were with transplant centers that were either in different countries, or in smaller hospitals that had less thorough or experienced transplant programs. Understanding the context of the information helped prepare me to compare apples to apples. Ultimately, there are never any guarantees, regardless of whether one uses the world's top surgeon and hospital. Yet, the track-record and quality of the transplant center can have a direct impact on patient outcomes and should be carefully considered.

Thus, after having time to process the positive and negative, I felt that I had collected enough information, answered many of my initial questions, and was finally deemed by the hospital as a "likely" candidate to donate.

Without making a decision or commitment to donate, I wanted to take the next step, move beyond the theoretical and find out how it was all relevant to me. I was pleased when Montefiore Medical Center invited me to continue my exploratory journey. In order to begin to weigh the decision, the conversation at this point would start to shift from whether or not I could donate, to what happens should I decide to donate.

I met with the transplant coordinator and was given a private seminar, complete with PowerPoint presentation to review all aspects of kidney donation. She told me all about kidneys, kidney disease, the medical statistics, the surgical options, risks and the recovery process. While much of the information was already familiar to me, I took copious notes and asked numerous questions. Hearing the information from the hospital's perspective helped me better understand the process and even picture myself going through it. This was a very empowering experience. Although I was far from ready to make a commitment, it helped give me the ability to begin considering a decision rooted in reality, and not based solely on information found on the Internet.

34. Why do I need a psychological evaluation?

Following my educational seminar, I recall feeling wonderful. I was fully aware of the great ability I had to now move forward and save someone else's life. However, it was at that point, that the hospital quickly put up a road block and brought me back down to reality, as the transplant coordinator then invited me to meet with a team of mental health professionals.

My first reaction was to be slightly offended. Here I am, doing such a wonderful thing and they had the *chutzpah* to suspect that I was not mentally sound! Not soon after the thought crossed my mind, did I realize how necessary this step was.

I was under the impression that since I was the one with the kidney to donate, the decision was mine alone to make. After all, the medical professionals had already concluded from a physical and medical perspective that I was a good candidate for donation. What more could anyone need?

But there is a good reason altruistic kidney donation is not common. For a person to willingly donate a kidney, they have to either be:

1. a deeply selfless person
2. coerced or bribed
3. suffering from mental illness

This is when I realized that, although there is a huge demand for kidney donors, hospitals are not desperate to take a kidney from anyone off the street willing to donate. Each and every transplant center is designed with multiple layers of protection to ensure the highest ethical standards are being met.

The last thing any hospital wants to do, is accept a kidney from someone who is not fully willing to donate, and perhaps is only doing so because they are being pressured, paid, or suffering from delusions that are compelling them to so. Such a violation of ethics would, not only put donors at risk, but compromise the integrity of the entire program and donation system. If that were to happen, all living-kidney donations would come to a screeching halt, and tens of thousands of recipients would be unable to receive urgently needed transplants. For that reason, the system is deliberately thorough, and each donor is put through a careful screening and interviews process, aimed at helping protect all the donors and recipients.

I first met with a psychologist who discussed my motives for wanting to donate. He was very complimentary and supportive but also was very helpful in playing devil's advocate. He raised many of the questions I had thought about and previously researched, such as whether I was familiar with the risks involved. Toward the end of our meeting, the psychologist dropped a question on me that I had not previously thought about, which really gave me pause. He asked, "how would you feel if you donated your kidney and a few days or weeks later, the kidney failed and the recipient was put back on the transplant list, or died?"

I sat back and thought about this question for a while. All of my previous considerations had weighed the risks to the donor against the benefit to the recipient. However, I had never really thought about what would happen if the donation failed. Essentially, this possibility would mean I had risked my life for nothing. Was that an outcome I was prepared to accept?

Over time, thinking about this question really gave me a new perspective. I slowly came to realize what real altruism is about. The act of helping another person wholeheartedly is not simply about doing so when the outcome is wonderful. It is about putting in one's own effort to do what is good, kind, just and helpful.

Having this counterbalance in my thought-process was very helpful, not only in ensuring I was fully informed, but bringing me to a deeper awareness of how I was evolving in my thinking. It helped me appreciate that I was undergoing my own personal transformation during this entire process. The more I understood and embraced the motivations behind my actions, the more confidently I was able to advance through this process.

35. Why do I need to meet with a social worker?

After meeting with the psychologist to confirm my mental fitness, I met with a physician to confirm my physical health. I then met with a surgeon to discuss my specific candidacy, and he walked me through every step of the surgery answering any questions I had. Overall, I was now deemed mentally and physically fit for the donation. However, I was both surprised and impressed when a social worker came to meet with me in order to discuss the bigger picture of my life.

She sat down and wanted to chat about my job and my family life. Initially, I thought she was simply being friendly and chatty. I quickly learned that this was yet another layer of the thorough process to protect donors. The social worker urged me to keep in mind that after the surgery, I was going to need a strong support system. I realized in that moment, that I had given so much thought to the surgery itself, I had neglected to think about who would be staying with me in the hospital, babysitting my children while I recuperate, driving carpool, taking down the garbage, or covering for me at work.

Since I am the type of person who always likes to be prepared, I found this part of the process to be a helpful one. It allowed me to take a step back and really think about all of the details of my daily life. Together, the social worker and I were able to brainstorm various scenarios that might come up, and review what my support system looks like, in order to see how all the gaps could best be filled. By asking these seemingly mundane questions, the social worker was able to help me put a practical plan into place to cover the daily components of my life, though basic, nevertheless, required careful thought and attention.

As kidney donors tend to be very generous people, they may not always put themselves first. Thus, by having honest conversations about their needs, it helps ensure that the donor is sufficiently prepared, protected and supported.

I recall one point during these conversations when I felt that these detailed discussions seemed very premature. After all, I had no concrete plans to donate, nor had I made a decision to do so. Why, then, would we be talking about who would be watching my kids while I recovered from surgery? The answer was quite simple. These conversations acted like a two-way street: It provided an opportunity for the transplant team to listen and learn more about me, so in the event I moved forward with the donation, they would be best poised to help me succeed. On the flip side, they were giving me as many tools and perspectives as possible to help me make my final decision, one based on truly comprehensive information and relevant to my own life.

36. What does the donor-advocate do?

After the hospital cleared me from a physical, mental and emotional standpoint, I soon learned that the donation itself was not fully cleared until a donor-advocate reviewed my candidacy. A donor-advocate is an independent physician, whose job is to equally examine my candidacy as a kidney donor, and to try and make a case as to why I should NOT donate a kidney. In other words, the donor-advocate acts as the "attorney" whose job it is to "defend" my health and my kidney and not rely on the hospital's assessment alone. Having a donor-advocate conduct a 360-degree analysis of my past, present and future health, adds another layer of protection to the well-being of the donor.

Why is this such a crucial step? Because let's be honest, even though the hospital has the best of intentions walking me through the kidney donation process, are they not somewhat biased? After all, the hospital is a business, and for both medical <u>and</u> financial reasons, the goal of their program is to transplant as many kidneys as possible. Their mission is certainly not to deter potential donors who are otherwise considering kidney donation.

Therefore, because there exists a conflict of interest, a donor should stop and ask whether the hospital is equally looking out for the donor, as they for themselves. It is for this reason that each donor is assigned a donor-advocate, which further helps protect the wellbeing and interests of the donor.

There are many donors who also opt to speak at length to their personal physician, to gain perspective from someone who is completely unrelated to the process and is familiar with his or her medical history.

37. How does the hospital make their final decision about my candidacy?

Although I was cleared as a likely candidate, I had not yet been approved. Once all of the medical data and information from my testing was collected, a meeting was scheduled for the entire team to discuss my candidacy. This meeting convened the surgeon, physician, transplant coordinator, psychologist, social worker and donor advocate to discuss all aspects of my case. Sitting around a table, they confidentially reviewed every aspect of my health and all the results of my tests and weighed the risks of donation.

This part of the process was not intended to be a mere rubber-stamping exercise, but rather, a thorough analysis of all the patient's information. Once all aspects of my physical, mental and emotional health were discussed and weighed, they collectively came to a conclusion - formally approving my candidacy for surgery.

In some instances, there may be a temporary reason for the team to decline a donor, such as obesity or high blood pressure. In these cases, the donor can either accept the information and forget about kidney donation, or choose to improve his or her own health, and then be reassessed at a later date. I have heard a number of stories of people who have lost in excess of 100 lbs. through diet and exercise to be a fit candidate for kidney donation. As a result, not only did they give life to someone else through their kidney donation, but they likely extended their lifespan by improving their own health.

It should be noted, if a person is rejected as a donor, he or she is entitled to get a second opinion by speaking to another hospital to help clarify or confirm the initial findings.

38. Can I speak to other donors to find out what their experience was like?

Absolutely! I found that speaking to other donors was one of the best ways to help allay the concerns I had. Nine out of ten times, donors had the most positive things to say about their experience. Don't get me wrong, surgery is not a walk in the park and many of the conversations gave me pause, or at least food for thought. In fact, I even encountered a number of websites dedicated to talking people out of donating their kidney. I carefully browsed and read them equally, as I sought to deepen my understanding of the challenges, risks and struggles of kidney donation.

Yet, since I was all about preparation, having people to speak to went a very long way. In fact, the donor community is a very strong and supportive network of people, who tend to be extremely caring and helpful to one another. There are a number of online discussion forums which not only provide helpful information, but offer to connect donors to those thinking about donation, so they can share their experiences and answer any questions.

39. Is my decision final, or can I change my mind later on?

Since the decision to donate belongs exclusively to the donor, he or she must be completely comfortable and can opt-out at any time in the process, without any recourse. Remember, just because a person is exploring this possibility, does not mean that they are obligated to donate.

However, some people tend to worry that once matched with a recipient, there is a sense of obligation to proceed with the donation, even if one is reluctant to go through with it. Nevertheless, a donor can back out at <u>any</u> point in the process, even as late as when they are getting onto the operating table. If a donor has a change of heart, he or she can always walk away. When I first heard this, I argued that it sounds good in theory, but in reality would not be easy to do. How could I live with the guilt of building up someone's hopes and then walking away? How can I do that to a recipient and just leave them hanging?

Once again, I was amazed at just how thoughtfully the system was setup to protect donors, even from feelings of guilt, shame and anxiety should they have a change of heart and decide to walk away. The transplant program will intervene on their behalf and explain to the recipient that due to new medical findings, the donor that had come forward is no longer a viable match for them.

Doing this helps protect donors by giving them the option to walk away at any point without suffering feelings of excessive guilt or obligation. It also helps the recipient move on and continue looking for a new kidney without any hard feelings. While the recipient may experience disappointment, he or she will likely also have feelings of hope, knowing there are donors out there who are trying to help and are willing to explore the possibility of kidney donation.

40. If I am matched, how soon will it be before the surgery?

When I began this process I feared, that as soon as I would be matched with a recipient, I would be whisked away to an operating table and find myself having surgery within 48 hours. I had envisioned a patient somewhere attached to a machine, fighting for life and would die within hours or days if not for this surgery. Perhaps it was my ignorance, or having watched too many movies that gave me this impression. This false perception created unnecessary anxiety for me.

In reality, patients in need of a kidney are desperately awaiting their transplant, however, they can often live for years with reduced kidney function. When the kidneys no longer do their job, patients are put on dialysis, which can further extend life for a number of years. Although dialysis is a temporary solution, it can often buy patients ample time for an ideal donor to be found and the surgery arranged.

Therefore, even when a suitable match is identified, there will be plenty of time to map out the process and arrange the many last details before undergoing surgery. In my case, nearly six-months passed between the time I was matched and the surgery itself. Having this larger window of time was very helpful for me to further process the enormity of my decision and to adequately make plans and arrangements to support an ideal recovery.

41. Can I push off the surgery for a more convenient time?

There was a point in time during my journey when I wrestled greatly with this question. On one hand, it was <u>my</u> kidney and I was constantly told by medical professionals I should not feel any pressure to donate. On the other hand, I knew there was a recipient somewhere who was suffering with each passing day while waiting for a kidney - their physical, mental, emotional and financial existence constantly being challenged - and I had the ability to alleviate their pain. Was it really appropriate for me to prolong the surgery for a few weeks or even a few months so it could be at a more convenient time for me?

From a medical perspective, I spoke to the transplant coordinator to better understand the risks to the recipient of delaying the surgery. I was told that in a case where the patient would soon need dialysis, but had not yet started treatments, it is often better for the recipient's health and medical outcome to undergo the transplant, prior to starting dialysis. However, if the recipient was already on dialysis, waiting a few extra months would not negatively impact the wellbeing or health of the recipient. While this is the general rule, each case should be evaluated individually, as in some circumstances the recipient may be in a more dire situation, with less time to wait.

From an ethical perspective, I struggled with the extent to which my delay would cause undo suffering to another person. After all, was my convenience (such as work or family schedule) a legitimate reason to extend another person's painful existence on dialysis?

To better work through my dilemma and uncertainty, I sought the guidance of medical experts, as well as faith leaders, and the feedback I received was consistent across the board. I was told that kidney donors must be given absolute flexibility, so they never feel as if they were being pressured into donating.

Additionally, if donors feel inconvenienced, they will be less likely to come forward to donate. If we lived in a world in which donors felt they did not have full control over their decision, it would negatively impact the entire "industry" and prevent others from donating in the future.

Once I had this knowledge, I was able to understand why there existed such a clear standard to protect donors from feeling any pressure. It was not only about protecting them and their kidney, but about protecting every future donor as well. The more the medical community goes above and beyond to protect donors, the more likely others will consider donation in the future. Therefore, as I began to make a more formal decision to move ahead with kidney donation, I did so with the knowledge that I would have time to properly plan for myself and my family - even though it meant delaying the surgery several months. Doing so allowed me to make all the arrangements necessary to support me through the surgery and recovery and help ensure the highest levels of success.

42. Can I delay the surgery until later in life?

Most people exploring kidney donation will quickly discover whether they are, or are not, a viable candidate for donation. However, there are often those who are a good candidate, but are not ready to donate (for a variety of personal reasons). If the timing is not right due to family, schooling, work, or even health issues - one could still proceed with kidney donation, albeit postpone the surgery for years or even decades later, until the time is right.

I have learned of donors who have undergone transplant surgery while they were in their sixties, seventies, and in a few rare cases, even their eighties! Therefore, if one conceptually feels that kidney donation speaks to them but faces a present conflict - instead of saying "no," one can simply say, "not now." Doing so keeps the option on the table and allows potential donors to step forward during another chapter of life. Keep in mind, however, that as one ages, new medical issues may arise that can potentially disqualify a person from being a kidney donor.

43. What if my remaining kidney fails and I need a kidney transplant in the future?

One of my major hesitations in proceeding with donation was out of concern I would be left with only one kidney. What happens if my remaining kidney fails, leaving me in urgent need of a transplant? Initially, it seemed foolish for me to donate a kidney, and leave myself so vulnerable. I would not have the "backup kidney" everyone else had, forcing me to go through the same long and painful process of waiting and looking for a donor. Imagine the irony if I gave my kidney to someone else, only to then need a transplant myself years later. This one frightening concern felt like enough of a reason to walk away from kidney donation.

However, I learned from a medical perspective, that the majority of patients who need a kidney are afflicted by kidney disease, a condition which equally attacks both kidneys at the same time. Thus, even when a person has two kidneys, this disease will still require the patient to receive a transplant and be put on the waiting list.

Additionally, I discovered that this concern was addressed by the many safety-measures built into the system of kidney donation aimed at protecting donors. Essentially, if a person who has donated a kidney then finds themselves in need of a kidney, they are automatically bumped up toward the top of the list and will be given priority above other recipients.

In other words, if a kidney donor and a non-kidney donor both needed a transplant, the kidney donor will likely receive a kidney more quickly than those on the waiting list that have two kidneys.

44. What if one of my children will need a kidney in the future?

Being a parent of four amazing kids, this concern felt very real. I understood the safety measure which protected donors, so that if I ever needed a kidney, I would move to the top of the list. However, the same would not be true if the child of a donor needed a kidney. Any parent would give a kidney to save the life of his or her own child without hesitation. Yet, as a kidney donor, I would be in a compromised position and unable to donate, as I would not have an extra one to give. Would it not make sense, therefore, to keep my kidney, just in case my child needed it in the future?

As I explored this very personal question more deeply, a number of factors helped give me clarity. First, I weighed the odds of anyone needing a kidney. As most people go through life without incident, I had no reason to suspect that any of my children would need a kidney transplant. However, if members of my family suffered from kidney issues or diabetes and had increased odds of needing a kidney, the decision would likely be a different one.

Second, I considered the fact that if by any remote chance one of my children ever needed a kidney, I was blessed with an amazing wife who would step up to donate without hesitation. Finally, even in the worst-case scenario, and I needed to ask friends, family, or community to consider donating, I already had the advantage of experience. Unlike other parents who advocate on behalf of their children, asking others to donate a kidney without having done it themselves, I would be in a unique position to speak about donation from firsthand experience. It would become a much easier "sell" to others, having done it myself - both from a physical and emotional standpoint. In other words, I would not be asking people to do something I myself would not do. Plus, as a donor, I enjoy the amazing moral support of so many people who truly admire donation and would step up to help, either by getting tested, or spreading the word to encourage others. Additionally, as a result of my donation, I have many relationships and connections to others throughout the nephrology community who could also offer guidance, contacts and support. All of these factors would give me an advantage over those who have not donated.

Keeping my kidney for a "rainy day" was a legitimate option. Certainly, in the event that someone I know or loved needed a kidney in the future, I would be glad I had not donated, as I would have the ability to help when they needed it most. Yet, it was a very theoretical long-shot - and even seemed silly, considering the fact there was a real person with a compelling need that could use a kidney today. This was an important struggle for me to endure, but, considering all of these factors, combined with my faith, I felt that donating my kidney to someone who needed it at the moment simply made the most sense to me.

Chapter 4.
The Fear of Telling Other People

45. How do I tell my spouse that I want to donate a kidney?

Prior to starting the formal testing, I had spent months thinking about and researching kidney donation, though it had been a private and deeply personal consideration. While I felt confident it was something I wanted to at least explore further, there was one small problem - I had not yet told my wife! I was quite concerned about how to drop this bombshell of a conversation on her, and I struggled to find the right way to bring it up. How does one tell their family that he or she is considering risking life and limb to help a total stranger?

Every family dynamic is different, and therefore, there is no single approach that works for everyone. When a friend or loved one is in need of a kidney, it is more understandable to raise the issue and tell a spouse that one is considering kidney. However, even under those circumstance, it is not uncommon for family members to have a negative reaction. In my situation, where my desire to donate was to a total stranger, it makes the conversation that much more difficult. Remember, potential donors may have been thinking about kidney donation for weeks or months. During that time donors strive to understand the process, struggle to reconcile the risks and challenges, and finally come to terms with them. Yet, for an unsuspecting family member, with one abrupt sentence the news can be dropped, altering their reality and giving them no time to process it. The jolt of such a revelation may leave them in a state of pure shock or even outrage.

Before beginning the conversation, it is important to recognize how unrealistic it is to expect family members to give a reasonable response, or pledge of support, without having the time to conduct the necessary research. It is advisable, therefore, to create a more slowly unfolding process and give them the opportunity to explore their own journey. This allows family members to absorb, process and struggle with the ideas and questions potential donors have already spent months thinking about and researching.

In preparing for the conversation with my wife, I was fairly sure I knew how it would go. As a husband and father of four young children, I was rather convinced my wife would tell me that kidney donation was completely out of the question, and more likely, that I was out of my mind.

Therefore, to soften what I anticipated being a brutal conversation, I invited my wife to go out to

Starbucks for a cup of coffee. Unsure of what her reaction would be, I nervously hoped that being in a public place would at least keep the conversation calm. Even as a therapist, I am a big believer in couples holding important conversations in environments which are optimistic and conducive to clear thinking and positive dialogue.

As we sat down and sipped our lattes, I explained that there was something on my mind I wanted her guidance on. I then took a deep breath and added, "but before I tell you what's on my mind, I am also going to make it easy and give you your response by telling you exactly what to say."

She looked at me with a very puzzled expression, but I nodded and just encouraged her to play along. I asked her to remember the following line and then play it back to me, "Ari, darling, sweetheart, I love you and you have a very generous heart, and I admire you for how giving you are, but with four young children at home now, this just is not the right time in our lives, and I think it would be best if you forget about this idea altogether."

I knew in my heart that if she only fed me this exact line, I would be done with the process. I could then put this entire silly idea behind me, for what I already knew was really a legitimate reason to not donate a kidney. This response would allow me to move on with my life, and still put my head on my pillow at night feeling good about myself for having tried to do a good deed.

Yet, she sat across the table staring at me. If she was not perplexed before, she now looked at me completely baffled. I smiled and asked her to please just remember her lines.

I took a deep breath and said to her that I was thinking about donating a kidney to save someone's life.

As the words came out of my mouth, I could only imagine how insanely ridiculous it sounded to her. Time stood still for a few moments as she processed what I had just told her. She then cleared her throat, leaned forward and said the following:

"Ari, darling, sweetheart, I love you and you have a very generous heart, and I admire you for how giving you are, but there are a million steps between wanting to donate a kidney and actually doing it. Therefore, instead of making the decision right now, why not just start the process of being tested. There is a good chance you may be disqualified due to a health reasons. But if you're not, and you successfully pass all the testing, we can then sit down and make the decision at that time."

While in hindsight, this was the most brilliant wisdom she could have possibly shared, at the time my jaw dropped open in shock and all I could respond was, "that was NOT your line!"

I was completely taken aback by her response. Not only was my wife incredibly supportive, but she helped me wrap my head around the enormity of this undertaking. She could not have been more accurate in giving me the guidance I needed.

Nobody can simply sit down over a cup of coffee and make such a major life choice. However, when broken down into a process, comprised of a series of small steps, it transformed a daunting decision into a more manageable one. That is exactly how I now approached this long road. My mindset shifted from struggling whether or not to donate a kidney, to learning if I was even a good candidate.

If I were to be rejected as a candidate, the decision would have been made for me and I would be able to move on with life. On the other hand, if I was deemed a great candidate, I would then be in a position to stop and think about making a decision that was based in reality, rather than theory.

My suggestion, therefore, to anyone looking to have this difficult conversation with a spouse, would be to start with my wife's approach. Rather than dropping the bomb on someone and frightening them with the news that you would like to donate a vital human organ, start with explaining you are interested in researching the topic and just exploring whether you are qualified to even consider it. All of this with the caveat that you are not rushing to make any decisions, only to become more educated about the topic.

46. How do I tell my children?

There are many circumstances in which children are subject to the decisions that parents make for them. In this situation, I wrestled with how and when to tell my kids. Was this a decision that required their "approval?" What if something went horribly wrong during the surgery? Would my children live with anger and resentment because their father voluntarily put himself at risk, placing another family before his own? Questions like this shook me to the core and I was unsure of how to proceed.

It's for this reason that my wife and I sat down with our children early on in this process to discuss it with them and gauge their reaction. Amongst ourselves, my wife and I decided that if for whatever reason our children were opposed to my kidney donation, we would abandon the process and return to our normal lives.

When we sat down to have this conversation, our two older children, Reuven and Meyer, were eleven and eight years old respectively, and our twins, Akiva and Aliza, were five. I began by explaining to them that everyone in life is given different strengths and weaknesses. I told them how some people have more, while others have less, yet, we are all given opportunities every day to help other people. I explained to them how the human body functions with the kidneys that we were born with. However, in the event that people do not have healthy kidneys, they are unable to live, unless someone comes forward to give one of his or her own kidneys as a gift.

I then told them that since I had two very healthy kidneys, I was thinking about possibly giving one to another person whose kidneys are sick and would die without receiving such a gift. Immediately my children began looking at me with frightened looks in their eyes. Meyer, my eight-year-old began crying. He explained to me that he thought it was a bad idea, as it sounded scary and was afraid of anything happening to me. I held my children as I wiped away their tears. I assured them that they did not have to be afraid, as I would not donate my kidney.

My wife and I then looked at each other as if we both understood that this would now be the end of the process. My son was right, it was not fair for me to risk my own life and put somebody else before our own family. Although a moment later, Reuven, my eleven years old turned to me and curiously asked, "well, who would you be giving your kidney to?"

I went on to tell them about a woman named Ronit who I was potentially paired with. He then asked if she had any children. I explained to my boys that she was a single mother who lived in Israel. She had three children at home and had been sick for many years and would not live much longer without a transplant.

My boys then looked at one another. Without uttering a word, they both nodded their heads yes. "In that case, we think that you should give her your kidney."

I found myself stunned and confused. I said to them, "hang on a second; a minute ago you told me that you did not want me to donate my kidney. Now you've changed your mind?!"

I tried explaining to them how the gravity of this decision was more than a simple yes or no question, such as, "would you like pizza for dinner?" This decision was permanent and life-changing, and not only for me.

Reuven then looked up at me with his big blue eyes and spoke words which felt as if they were divinely inspired. When we heard them, my wife and I both knew that we were making the right decision. He said, "if you have the surgery and anything bad happens to you, we will be very sad, but at least we will have mommy to take care of us. But if this lady does not receive the kidney, she will die, and her children will be left as orphans. For that reason, you should give her your kidney."

The room was silent as it reverberated with his innocence, compassion and wisdom. Not only did that moment give us the clarity that we were seeking in this entire process, but it blew me away to appreciate that this decision was not only going to impact the recipient, however, my own children would forever be transformed as well. In the process, their lives, too, were being changed, as they were developing a mature sense of empathy and altruism to care for the plight of other people.

This one conversation completely shifted how I was progressing through the process. No longer was it only about me or a surgery, but it was an exercise in understanding our children, our approach to parenting, and our family's values and priorities. It became something that would strengthen our family and hopefully inspire our children throughout the rest of their lives. Instead of my children being a barrier to the process, as I had initially expected, they ultimately became the drive and motivation to give me the confidence I needed to progress further on my journey.

47. How do I tell my parents?

Often, when adults speak to their parents, they regress into an earlier childhood version of themselves. This is particularly true when discussing major life decisions. As adults, even though parental approval is no longer needed, grown children still long for their parent's acceptance.

Therefore, before I was able to present the idea of kidney donation to my parents, I spent many hours thinking about how that conversation might go. I nervously played it over in my head again and again and practiced the answers to the questions they would ask. However, I was overlooking one major issue.

While I had invested months into the exploration of kidney donation, and my mind had searched for all of the intellectual answers to satisfy my curiosity and concern, for a parent, the issue is far more of an emotional exercise than an intellectual one.

I neglected to consider, that despite the hundreds of hours I had spent researching and learning about kidney donation, a parent is only focused on one issue - keeping their children safe. The reality is, whether one is a parent of a five-year-old, or a forty-five-year-old, they constantly worry about their child's safety and well-being. Although I was blessed with parents who have always supported and encouraged me and helped shape me into the person I am today, I was not prepared for the resistance I would face when I told them I was voluntarily putting myself at risk.

Similarly, I am sure that any child who proudly tells their parents that they are joining the military, becoming a firefighter or police officer expects a pat on the back and tremendous kudos. After all, making such a selfless commitment to help other people seems like a positive reflection on the very parents who nurtured and raised such a caring and compassionate child. However, one should not confuse a parent's fear with their lack of pride. Simply because a parent is terrified to lose their child does not mean they are not proud. It simply means they are doing their job as a parent to protect their beloved child. This was my exact experience.

Knowing that my mother had spent decades working in a hospital, I contextualized the conversation through the lens of medicine. I explained to my mother that I had recently become aware of something she encounters everyday - people struggling with medical hardships. I explained that I had been doing months of research to learn about people with kidney disease and what could be done to help them.

Ultimately, the conversation shifted to my interest in actually donating one of my kidneys. While my mother was extremely concerned, coming from a medical background, we spent a bulk of the conversation discussing the medical side of the process. While she was rightfully skeptical, her main concern was that I do my homework to really learn everything I could about the short and long-term risks of the surgery and life with only one kidney. She helped me consider new questions I had not previously entertained and urged me to find the answers before making any decisions. There is no doubt she was filled with mixed emotions - somewhere between proud and terrified - but she was overall very supportive. In particular, it was helpful for me to convey to my mother that I had not yet made any decisions, but was simply being tested and giving the topic consideration.

The conversation with my father, however, was far more sobering. Being a thoughtful and risk-averse person (who also dislikes hospitals), he was neither interested in hearing all of my well-rehearsed answers about the medical side, nor was he interested in being convinced that his son's life should be put in any unnecessary danger.

Was he wrong? Absolutely not.

However, after making his opposition very clear to me, I realized that I was in a very difficult position. Although I am an adult who has the right to make my own decisions, I had no intention of blatantly defying my father's will, or disrespecting his wishes. Yet, I still felt very strongly about continuing the process. I felt it was my parents who raised me to be a considerate and caring person, and, thus, I was very torn about what to do next.

Therefore, I put myself in my father's shoes. I began to think about how I would react if one of my children were to come to me and make the same case. I recognized that even with all my newly acquired knowledge on the topic of kidney donation, as a parent, I would likely express the exact same opposition as my father. After all, from the moment our children are born, our entire existence is dedicated to trying to keep them safe and healthy. How could I, therefore, permit my child to risk his or her own life?

With this new perspective I was able to really appreciate where my father was coming from. It enabled me to revisit the conversation with him, albeit, seeing it now through his eyes. I shared with him that I had come to see and understand his perspective and really appreciated his concerns.

It was this realization that allowed me to find the right words I was looking for. It helped me realize that I was neither approaching him to ask for his approval or his blessing to donate a kidney. Rather I was coming to him to ask for his understanding and support during the process, even though he did not agree with the decision.

This shift in perspective was a major turning point. My father paused for what felt like an eternity and said the following, "I really don't like what you're doing and I do not approve of my children putting themselves at risk. However, I'm very proud of you and will be by your side to help you throughout the process."

I was truly blown away by my father's response and I appreciated how difficult it must have been to arrive at that conclusion. I learned from this, that while having one's family offer both approval <u>and</u> support is ideal, sometimes one can only reasonably ask for their support and welcome their love, even if it does not come with their full approval.

48. How do I tell my employer?

There are generally two concerns an employer may have regarding kidney donation. The first, and more common concern, is the void one will leave when taking time off from work during the surgery and recovery. The second, and more personal concern, is for the welfare and health of the employee in light of such a major life-decision. It is important, however, that the two areas of concern not be confused.

Although most employers care greatly about the well-being of their employees, their primary obligation is to run an efficient and productive business. Therefore, if and when the time is right for a person to tell their employer about their plan to donate a kidney, it may be a good idea for an employee to begin by providing immediate reassurance that he or she will not take an abrupt medical leave without first arranging proper coverage. Because there will be ample time to make arrangements, one's supervisor or boss can be easily included in the planning process so it does not create a professional hardship, nor jeopardize one's employment.

In my case, I was particularly nervous to break the news to my employer, as I worked as a full time rabbi, ministering to hundreds of families who relied upon me for many spiritual, educational and pastoral needs. I knew my community would be filled with a range of mixed responses to my desire to donate a kidney, including concerns for both my health and time away from work.

When word spread throughout the community, most people were supportive, while many were deeply concerned for my well-being. I, therefore, proposed a plan to have my professional responsibilities covered while I was recuperating. Additionally, I proposed that the congregation allow me 2 weeks of unpaid leave in order to recover, followed by another week, where I would be allowed to return to work on a part-time basis as I fully regained my strength. Yet, despite the mixed responses, I quickly learned how blessed I was. Proud of my commitment to help others, the congregation's leadership had voted to give me 4 complete weeks of vacation and they insisted on paying me my full salary while I recuperated. Needless to say, I was extremely touched by the gesture and the outpouring of support.

While every person has a unique arrangement and relationship with their employer, some will offer kidney donors paid time off, others will provide unpaid leave for the duration the surgery and recovery, while most will encourage their employees to use their sick leave and vacation days for the surgery and recovery. Once again, I will reiterate that a donor may not receive any form of compensation for donating a kidney. At the same time, this generous deed should not cost donors money or a loss of wages. Therefore, if an employer is unable to cover the salary during the process, there may be charitable foundations and organizations which can offer lost-wage reimbursements so donors do not lose money or feel a disincentive to donate.

It is best for one to be thorough in researching their benefits and have an honest conversation with a supervisor, laying out the time frame for how long one will be out of work, and when he or she plans to return. Federal employees may discover they are granted 30 days of paid time off for organ donation, and each State will have their own regulations for organ-donor benefits. Additionally, one should keep in mind that returning to work need not be all or nothing. Though I was unable to return to work right away, just a few days after surgery I was able to spend a several hours each day on the computer, responding to emails and conducting some light business. Through open conversations, one can work collaboratively to explore the perfect balance that works best for the donor and the employer.

49. How do I respond to people who tell me I'm crazy?

While the vast number of comments I received were largely positive statements of support from friends and family, there were also negative comments that I had to deal with. Such comments brought a wave of mixed emotions, and at times, I found them hurtful. After all, I was pushing myself to find the inner strength to do something incredible, and I was now forced to not only confront my personal struggle, but to also wrestle with the criticism of others.

It took me some time to step back and understand how to process the negative comments. First, I had to realize that what felt like criticism was actually coming from a place of love, as they were coming from people who were not trying to be hurtful. On the contrary, these people cared for me but were not able to find kind words to express their concern.

Moreover, I eventually realized calling me "crazy" was not actually wrong. "Crazy" is the word people use as an adjective for something they think is not normative. The truth is, to even consider kidney donation, one already stands out of the crowd, or as some might put it, seem a little "crazy." Although they may have been critical, I soon learned that what they were actually saying was, "kidney donation is incredible, but it is something that I could never do."

It took me some time, but I eventually grew more comfortable with the idea that not everyone viewed life as I did. It did not mean I was "crazy," but it certainly meant I was different than others around me, and that was something I was happy to accept. This nuance further emphasizes why it is important to never pressure someone to donate. For even if one person views the kidney-donation process as a very straightforward road, most others will view it differently.

While it would behoove all members of society to offer support and gratitude for those who make personal sacrifices for the greater good, it is unrealistic to expect such an optimistic response. Thus, instead of responding to people who were critical of my interest in kidney donation, I learned to simply smile and listen while nodding my head and thank them for their concern and ask them to keep me in their prayers. Since my entire journey was an extremely personal one, it was neither my goal nor responsibility to try and convince others it was the right decision. The important point was that it was the right decision for me.

50. I am hesitant to tell people, should I keep my kidney donation a secret?

This was another very personal struggle for me. Because I spent so many months thinking about kidney donation without having made a final decision, it was difficult for me to explain and justify my rationale to others in a mere sentence or two. I found that the more people I told, the more I would have to go on the defensive and explain to others what I was thinking and feeling. Therefore, I quickly learned that during the early part of the process and testing phase, it was easier to not share my journey with others, outside of my inner circle of close family and friends. This allowed me to continue the private exploration, without welcoming opinions from others, regarding a topic I myself had not personally made a final decision about.

However, there was a turning point in the process when that changed. As I made the decision to proceed with the actual transplant, I wanted the support of others in my community. I no longer wanted to go through this journey alone and in secrecy. It was at that point in time I was far more open and expressive about donation and was comfortable asking others for their prayers and support, which they always pledged willingly.

I noticed, however, that for months following my successful kidney donation, I was again hesitant to speak out or discuss it with other people. I feared others might see it as though I were bragging and showing off to the world what a saintly person I was. This fear caused me to remain silent and humble.

The initial part of the journey was very much about me. It was a process of personal transformation to push myself to new limits and explore how far I would go to make an impact on the world. However, even after I had completed my donation, I found myself questioning what else I could do to help those still suffering with kidney disease. I soon realized that the 4 million other kidney patients around the world who were still waiting for a kidney could be helped if I spoke out and shared my story. While it took me time to overcome my shyness about talking openly on this very private topic, I knew that in addition to donating my kidney, I still had the ability to continue saving lives by simply speaking up.

So, I eventually learned to once again speak out and share my story. The more people knew about my donation, the more likely they would be to consider, explore or promote kidney donation, or at least support others thinking about starting their own journey.

Chapter 5.
The Surgery

51. What is the difference between a laparoscopic and open surgery?

Historically, abdominal surgeries required an extensive incision to remove the kidney. This type of open-procedure took a longer amount of time to recuperate, left a more visible scar, and had increased odds of certain complications. However, today, the process of removing a kidney is usually done laparoscopically. A laparoscopic surgery is an amazing way to remove a kidney without having to fully open the donor's abdomen.

In a laparoscopic procedure, the surgeon makes two small incisions (each about one inch long) and uses specialized tools to insert into these sites to maneuver inside the abdomen. Using tiny cameras that are attached to the laparoscopes, the kidney can be secured and removed from the abdomen through a third incision site. The third incision is also small - usually less than 3 inches in length - and is made along the belly button where the scar will be well blended and hidden.

The advances in surgical technology are amazing. Any woman who has ever given birth by C-section knows the difficulties involved in recuperating from a full open incision. It can be a slow and often painful experience. However, with a laparoscopic procedure, the surgery itself is quicker, and has a much faster and less painful recovery time.

52. Are there any additional risks?

As with all surgeries, there is a "laundry" list of potential complications and risks. When I first read through the extensive list I felt highly discouraged. However, like warning labels on any box of cold medicine, I wondered whether the concerns were "real" or simply legal disclaimers to prevent liability in the remote chance something goes wrong.

As consumers we don't only weigh the risks, but the likelihood of the risks against the benefits. Let's be honest, if a possible side-effect of taking Advil is that it can lead to a stroke, why would anyone ever take this medication? Would a person not prefer to have a mild headache than accept the risk of having a stroke? But because the chance of a stroke is so remote, most people are willing to take those chances and pop a few Advil when they have a headache. The risks are, nevertheless, printed on the package because there have been documented cases of catastrophic side-effects. When one makes a decision to take any medication, it is a decision to take a chance and hope they are not in the minority of people who suffer such side-effects.

Surgery is the same. There are countless risks one should carefully review, consider and weigh, regardless of their likelihood. For me, as a frequent traveler, I thought about the many flights I have taken. Without exception, each flight began with showing me how to inflate my life-jacket in the "unlikely event of a water landing." Yet, have I ever had to inflate my life-jacket? Of course not. The majority of people who fly will never require a life-jacket. But, as means of being prepared and informed, the industry standard is to notify travelers of potential risks and how to best handle them.

While the list of complications is long, with kidney donation, the most common side effect is developing an infection at the incision site, which if it occurs, would be treated with antibiotics. The surgeon also informs donors about the possibility of a "conversion," although it is unlikely. This is when during a laparoscopic procedure, the doctors notice a complication which requires them to open the patient's abdomen in order to safely complete the procedure.

I found the scariest part of weighing these risks was the notion of permanence. In some cases, donors may forever live with chronic pain or discomfort, and other serious complications can even lead to death. I spent considerable time not only weighing the risks, but asking myself what the value was in my own existence, and measuring the extent I was willing to go to save a life.

While the complications are highly unlikely, the doctors will discuss them with donors, so they can consider all the facts when making the decision and be more likely to take precautionary steps to help reduce the odds of problems arising. I continually reminded myself throughout the process that any outcome was, in fact, a possibility. However, just as flying, driving, or crossing the street involves some level of risk, each person should make a careful calculation regarding the amount of risk they are comfortable taking. This is a very personal reckoning, and one should not feel any pressure to make a decision that does not fit who they are.

53. Is there anything I can do to help the success of the surgery and recovery?

Kidney donation has become somewhat routine, and the risks well known, but there are still things that can be done to improve the overall outcome.

Personally, I took great pride in knowing I was in good enough health to be selected as a candidate for kidney donation. However, when being completely honest with myself, I knew I could be healthier and even afford to lose an extra 30 lbs.

Therefore, I used this journey as an opportunity to challenge and transform myself. I began to diet and joined a gym, working out several times per week. I focused on jogging and running, so I could improve my cardiovascular functioning. This would help my heart and lungs grow stronger, which would support better outcomes during the surgery and recovery. I also did a great deal of stretching, especially to improve my flexibility and side to side mobility. This was done with the intention of reducing the soreness that some people report following hours of being on an operating table.

I am glad to report that my heart and lungs did great during the surgery and recovery, and I had no soreness at all in my back. Was it related to my exercise and stretching? I can't be sure, but I would like to think it helped.

Another benefit to my exercise routine was discovering strength I never knew I had. I am not referring to my physical strength, but to my mental abilities. There were numerous times when I found myself running on the treadmill, and my body wanted to simply quit. I was sweating, tired and out of breath. However, I was surprisingly able to push my mind to keep going. Regardless of the level of challenge, or even the pain I felt while running, I learned to find purpose in every step, which propelled me to push harder and keep going. In my heart, I knew that every step I took would help me grow stronger. I knew that it would provide a leaner, less fatty, and healthier kidney to give to Ronit. It was that sense of purpose, which motivated me to push myself on a deeper level than ever before and achieve new things I previously would not have been able to do.

This mindset also proved to be a valuable mental tool I employed during the recovery process, because when I experienced any pain or discomfort following surgery, I was better prepared to handle it. After having spent months on the treadmill learning to push beyond the pain or fatigue, I felt as if my threshold for discomfort had increased, helping me to become more fully prepared physically, emotionally and psychologically. My mind was now trained to recognize discomfort, but not let it stop me.

As a result of this newfound determination, I managed to lose 30 lbs. and get in the best shape of my life. This is yet, another example of how I benefited, transformed, and learned more about myself, from the process of kidney donation.

54. Will I meet the recipient?

When one donates a kidney to a friend or family member, they obviously already have a relationship.

However, for altruistic donors who give to a total stranger, many will opt to never meet the recipient. Thus, they may choose to not reveal themselves, but to maintain their anonymity. Perhaps this is due to a strong sense of humility surrounding their donation. Such donors are the ones who never wish to receive a word of gratitude, and instead perform this incredibly generous act of kindness, without any recognition at all.

Other altruistic donors may choose to remain anonymous because of an inner fear. What might happen if they met the recipient prior to the transplant, but felt they simply did not like the person? What would they do next? Would the donor continue and donate to someone they were uncomfortable with? Would they choose someone else and live with the guilt of disappointing the first person? Or perhaps, would they walk away from donation altogether? Regardless of the choice, meeting a recipient can potentially create a very uncomfortable experience, which could be avoided simply by not meeting. Other donors will choose to not meet their recipient until weeks, months or years following the donation.

However, in my situation, I was very happy to meet my recipient in advance and was glad I did! Being the positive person I am - one who always looks for the good in others - I was confident and hopeful I would form a meaningful connection with my recipient.

In the week prior to surgery I was invited to the hospital for a final round of pre-op testing. After the blood tests were completed, the transplant coordinator told me that the recipient was also in the hospital going through a final round of testing, and asked if I was interested in meeting her. After excitedly agreeing, I was taken into the hospital chapel, where I met Ronit for the first time.

With her teenage daughter standing at her side, Ronit stood up to greet me and the room was immediately filled with overflowing emotion. Though I was unsure of how to initially react, I noticed through their sobs and tears they were both smiling from ear to ear. It is simply beyond description to explain the joy that was exuded. Ronit stepped forward as she wiped away her tears and tried to catch her breath. In a humble, soft and broken voice, all she kept

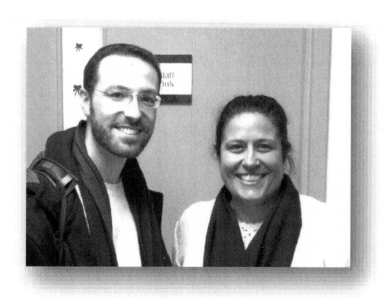

saying to me was, "thank you, thank you, thank you." It was at that moment, as chills ran up my spine that I began to realize the true impact my decision was having.

Ronit was no longer a case or a file, she was a real person with a real family. It was incredible to look into her eyes and to begin understanding the piece of the puzzle that was missing from this year-long journey. It was at that moment I started to truly get it. Even after having spent so much time researching, learning and testing, I realized that until I looked into the eyes of the recipient, someone so desperate for a chance to live, I could not possibly fully understand what kidney donation was about.

I knew that from my perspective, the process of kidney donation would involve some risk, discomfort, and perhaps inconvenience. But how could I weigh that against what it meant for Ronit? After meeting her, I understood just how badly she wanted a chance at life, and my five-ounce kidney was the difference between life and death.

Although I fully respect each donor's decision whether or to meet their recipient, from my own experience, I was only too glad to have taken the time to have met my recipient. It helped me continue my journey with an even greater commitment and understanding of what the journey was about. Today, even years later, our families are close and not a week goes by when I don't receive a beautiful email from Ronit. Having that life-long connection to her is truly remarkable!

55. Is there anything specific I should bring to the hospital?

In keeping to my theme of doing everything in my power to be completely prepared, I wanted to bring anything to the hospital that would give me any advantage during my stay. However, the truth is, the hospital provided me everything I needed.

However, there were several items which I did not technically need, but were helpful in adding to my own comfort, even in the smallest ways. I brought an extra-soft pillow from home to help me get more comfortable at night. I brought an iPad loaded with books and videos, so if I could not sleep, I would not have to worry about flipping through channels and searching for something to help me pass the time, because I could immediately watch what I enjoyed. I even made a special playlist of music I could listen to when I wanted to relax, and another high-energy playlist to keep me motivated for my post-surgery walks around the hospital.

My wife got a particular kick out of watching me walk laps around the hospital floor on the day following surgery. I put in my earbuds and listened to the exact same music I played one week earlier as I ferociously ran a seve-minute mile on the treadmill. Yet, this time, as the high-intensity music played and my mind was running a seven-minute mile, my feet were ever so slowly shuffling on the floor - step, step, pause, repeat. Personally, I found the music to be a great motivator to push me to continue walking, even when I felt like going back to bed.

While none of these "extras" were necessary to bring to the hospital, for many donors, it can be the little things that make the difference in helping them feel that much more comfortable.

56. Will I have to wear one of *those* gowns?

Although I was hoping to be the exception, the answer to this one was quite clear (literally). Yes, every patient has to wear one of those revealing hospital gowns. However, there are two very important things to note about these gowns.

The first is that they provide little dignity. As a result, no matter how many ways I tried to tie those strings, the gown would not quite do what I wanted. One can always ask for a second gown, and wear one in the front and one in the back to feel a little more dignified. However, I have learned to appreciate that there is a symbolic rite of passage to wearing the infamous hospital gown. It represents that critical shift - where a patient stops taking themselves too seriously, and instead, embraces their "sheer" humanity and frailty. The quicker this process happens, the quicker the patient can sit back and not even think about it. Instead of one constantly fighting the blankets to cover up and feel dignified, the gown empowers an incredible sense of personal liberation, where patients quickly learn to own their reality, and not care about what others think.

The second benefit of the gown, is a very practical one. After having abdominal surgery, I was most comfortable when nothing touched or pressed directly on my stomach. Therefore, the hospital gowns were the perfect and most comfortable attire imaginable. In fact, when it was time to leave the hospital, I had brought a rather stretchy pair of sweat pants to wear. However, while they were loose fitting, they were nowhere nearly as comfortable as the hospital gown. Needless to say, I was somewhat disappointed when the nurse declined my request to take my comfortable and beloved hospital gown home with me.

57. Will I have to have a urinary catheter?

While on the topic of putting one's dignity aside, let's candidly cover the topic of the catheter. The answer is yes, every surgical patient receives a urinary catheter, which is a small tube placed in the urethra and collects urine so one does not need to go to the bathroom.

In my research I learned I was not alone in my fear of having a urinary catheter, as many people expressed concerns about this one specific component of the surgery. In fact, I will admit there were times during this process when I was so uncomfortable with the idea of having a catheter, that I halted my research and stopped considering kidney donation for months. While it may seem like such a small part of the overall picture, for me, and many others, it was a big deal.

Medically speaking, the catheter plays an important role. After a kidney is removed, the second kidney must kick into overdrive and adapt to its new job of singlehandedly producing all the body's urine, which it miraculously does. What doctors expect to see immediately following surgery is a decrease in one's urine output, followed by a healthy surge. Thus, in order to protect the remaining kidney during this transition, the patient receives plenty of IV fluids which keeps the body and the kidney very well hydrated and healthy. As a result, the kidney can get right to work processing the additional fluids. Having a urinary catheter is the perfect way for the doctors to directly measure the urine output and be sure the remaining kidney is doing its job as expected.

While the mere thought of the urinary catheter provided me with anxieties and fears, these concerns were quickly allayed at various stages of the surgery and recovery.

1. The catheter was placed while I was already under anesthesia and fast asleep. This may be a huge relief for people struggling with the thought of how uncomfortable it would seem to have it placed while awake. For me, when I woke up from surgery, it was just there and I was a happy camper.

2. Having the catheter helped me avoid post-surgical pain. I recall the feeling after surgery, when I was exhausted and resting to regain my strength, and I had a random thought pass through my mind. I considered just how dreadful it would be if I had to get myself out of bed just to go use the bathroom. I was surprised at myself for being so happy to have the catheter and to not have to even think about getting up. In the end, the catheter was a "lifesaver" and I was so glad to have it!

3. Removing the catheter was not as awkward as I expected. On the day following surgery patients are encouraged to walk around. This meant it was time for the catheter to be removed. This was the part I was dreading the most. Would it be painful? Would it be awkward? I just was not sure what to expect.

    Call me immature, but my first moment of relief came when the person who entered my room to remove the catheter was a male nurse. In my curious style, I asked him to explain exactly what happens and what to expect. The nurse was very patient, helpful and really put me at ease. He told me it would not hurt at all, rather, it would just be a strange sensation, similar to the feeling of urinating. Best of all, it would be very quick.

I appreciated that the nurse kept me covered the entire time and explained what he was doing as he was doing it. Before I knew it, he was done - there was no pain, and the actual removal of the catheter took less than two seconds. I could not believe how nervous I was for something so simple! Honestly, I've gotten haircuts that were more traumatic!

It is interesting that what I feared the most was actually the least significant part of the entire process.

58. What can I eat prior to the surgery?

From midnight the night before surgery, the doctors instruct patients to not eat or drink anything. This is because they want patients to have an empty stomach during the surgery to avoid complications under anesthesia. However, the day prior to the surgery, one can eat as they normally would.

Personally, I tried to keep it light, knowing I wanted my stomach and digestive tract to feel calm and not stressed going into the surgery.

59. What happens when I arrive at the hospital?

For many donors, this is where things start to get "real." However, I was not so much nervous or anxious, as much as curious. There tends to be two types of patients: the ones who look away when they get a blood test, and the ones who want to watch. There are those who want to understand the ins and outs of a procedure and have a doctor explain what is happening at each moment, and there are those who would rather not know the details and simply say, "just tell me when you're done."

I learned during this entire process that I am the former. I took comfort in knowing what to expect and wanted to know what would be happening at every turn. I appreciated that the transplant coordinator was extremely patient and helpful in making sure all of my questions were answered. I was given very clear instructions about when to arrive at the hospital, where to park my car and exactly where to go. To my surprise, when I arrived in the pre-op area, the room was filled with great energy and excitement. There were lots of hugs, group photos and, of course, tons of paperwork.

While forms and paperwork are part of every hospital stay, in the case of someone voluntarily undergoing an elective procedure for the benefit of another person, it can be even more extensive, as they want to be sure kidney donors are proceeding of their own volition and without any pressure or coercion. Since it had been months leading up to this point, the paperwork did not surprise me. I remember holding the pen in my hand, and with each document I signed, I felt a sobering feeling. More significant than acknowledging the legalities of the paperwork, putting my signature on those papers was an affirmation of my identity - it reflected my name, my signature and my choice.

Even while checking into the hospital I felt calm. I still knew I could walk away at any moment without any recourse and I took pride in each signature I penned, knowing it was a way for me to stand by my decision.

After the paperwork, I was brought to the pre-op waiting room, where I was given the famous set of gowns to change into. My wife took the bag containing my clothes, and I sat comfortably on the bed. Just several feet away from me, sitting on the other side of the curtain was my kidney recipient, Ronit. She was being prepped for her surgery, which would take place in a parallel operating room, so immediately after my kidney was removed, it could be quickly transplanted into her abdomen.

My wife and I sat calmly, joking around and enjoying the quiet, when we noticed the sound of crying coming from beyond the curtain. My wife called out with the words, "knock- knock" and asked Ronit if everything was OK. As she peeked her head into Ronit's side of the curtain, my wife saw Ronit sobbing against her teenage daughter's chest. My wife walked over and joined in the group hug and again asked if Ronit was OK.

Ronit responded, "I could not be better. Please don't misunderstand me. These are tears of pure joy! I have waited for years to find a kidney, but I thought I would leave this world and leave my children before ever finding someone so generous. I just can't believe this day is here and I am so overjoyed it is actually happening."

While I sat on the bed, waiting for the doctors to come in and talk to us before the surgery, I felt so blessed to have heard those incredible words from Ronit and to appreciate the depths of her raw emotion. What a powerful reminder of what I was doing and why I was doing it! I smiled as I further reflected how the journey had never really been about the surgery, the extra pillows, playlists, iPad or any of the other forms of preparation upon which I had been focusing - this was all about the precious value of saving a human life.

60. When will they wheel me into the operating room?

Surprisingly, was not wheeled into the operating room. I had always pictured myself laying comfortably on a bed with pillows and blankets and being wheeled into the operating room, comfortably drugged. I found it to be a very strange feeling when it was time for surgery and the nurse invited me to say goodbye to my family and follow her into the operating room.

I later learned that for most surgeries a patient is wheeled into the operating room. However, for kidney donation, donors are typically asked to walk themselves in and climb up onto the operating table. This allows donors another opportunity to say, "no thanks, I've actually changed my mind and don't want to go through with it." If the hospital were to wheel donors into the operating room, it would literally and figuratively seem as if they were "pushing" them into it. Therefore, beyond having signed all of the paperwork agreeing to the surgery, to emphasize the autonomy and free will of the donors, they are asked to walk themselves into the operating room and make a physical gesture of their decision to proceed with the transplant.

61. How long does the surgery last?

The surgery lasts on average between 2-3 hours. Often doctors will predict a longer completion time, so the family should not worry in the event the surgery takes longer. This gives the surgeons the opportunity to pleasantly surprise the family and let them know they finished ahead of schedule. While they certainly do not rush the procedure, the doctors also do not wish to keep a patient under anesthesia longer than necessary, as it could increase risk factors. This is why they are mindful of the time and will stay in constant communication with family members before, during and after the surgery.

62. What actually happens during the surgery?

While the surgery itself begins the anesthesia, which puts the patient into a nice deep sleep, a sedative can be administered through the IV to help the patient feel more relaxed upon entering the operating room.

I recall laying on the operating table, chatting and joking with the nurses and doctors. As the room is bright and quite cold, the nurses offered to cover me with some warm blankets that had been heated up. Enjoying the blankets, combined with the sedative I was given through the IV, I quickly felt very relaxed, drowsy and even loopy. I continued chatting and joking around, until it was time for the anesthesia. I asked for a moment to recite a personal prayer. As a spiritual person, I took advantage of this opportunity and asked God to watch over me and Ronit, and guide the hands of the surgeons to operate successfully. I felt a great sense of peace, knowing I had done everything in my power to arrive safely at this point, and the rest was out of my hands. This prayer allowed me to express that feeling in a meaningful way.

I was then given the anesthesia and quickly drifted into a deep a sleep.

There are two versions of what happened next, my conscious reality, and what was actually taking place.

As far as my conscious reality was concerned, I was given the oxygen mask and asked to take a few deep breaths to allow the anesthesia to do its job. I then fell into an amazing deep sleep, only to wake up in what felt like a moment later. In my conscious reality, I took a nap, woke up and found myself in the recovery room. In fact, I remember asking myself when I woke up why was the surgery not done? After all, it seemed as if I had just dozed off briefly, and I woke up feeling fine, yet, very sleepy. As far as I was concerned, it all just felt like a quick nap. It was hard to believe that it was over in the blink of an eye.

Then there was the other part of the story - the actual reality of what took place during those few hours.

After the anesthesiologist put me "under," a breathing tube was placed in my throat in order to protect my airway. I was told to expect that I may have a dry or sore throat as a result of the breathing tube. However, I was glad that I experienced neither. In fact, I would not have even known a tube had been placed had they not told me about it.

During the laparoscopic procedure, the doctors made 2 small incisions (about an inch wide) to insert the laparoscopes. Even though the wand-like scopes have cameras and lights on them, to maximize the field of view and best see what they are doing, doctors inflated my abdomen with air. Then, by maneuvering the two wands, almost like robotic hands, they were able to conduct the surgery with minimal trauma to my body. The doctors then removed my kidney from what they call a "keyhole incision," which they neatly made around the bellybutton. As the kidney is smaller than the size of an average fist, it was then removed by rotating it lengthwise and passing it through the keyhole incision which was only 2-3 inches wide.

The three small incisions were then closed with a few stitches and covered in steri-strip bandages. That was it. After waking from anesthesia, my bed was wheeled into the recovery room, where I was monitored more closely for the initial few hours after surgery.

63. Where does the recipient's surgery take place?

Shortly after my surgery had started, Ronit's began in an adjacent operating room,. Once my kidney was removed, it was walked next door and surgically placed into her abdomen. I was told that literally within minutes of attaching the kidney, the doctors watched as it produced healthy urine. This was the first time in years that Ronit's body was able to do so, and the first sign the surgery was a success.

64. Where will my family be during the surgery?

I was glad my wife was able to stay with me right up until it was time for me to enter the operating room, at which point she went to the waiting room. For me, I had the "easy" part, as I just slept through it. For her those few hours were long. The doctors provided reports during the surgery to keep my wife updated and to give her the peace of mind that everything was going smoothly.

Once I was in the recovery room, my wife was able to come and see me. Although I felt very drowsy, I was still smiling, talking and even joking around.

65. Will surgery be painful?

Like many people on this journey, this was definitely one of my biggest concerns. As some people have higher pain thresholds and would be willing to tolerate a more painful experience, others would opt-out if they knew the pain would be beyond their comfort zone. For that reason, I felt it was important to know in advance what to expect.

Personally, I am someone that has a rather low threshold for pain. As may be stereotypical of many men, when I have a headache, I am the person who wants to climb back into bed. Therefore, I was rather concerned about how I would handle the pain following abdominal surgery. However, I am glad to report that, while surgery is serious and not a walk in the park, there was never a moment throughout the journey during which I felt any excruciating pain. Sure, there were certainly moments of discomfort which came and went in varying degrees and durations. At no point, though, did it reach a level which made me question whether I made a mistake. The pain-management team, led by the anesthesiologist, was great at making sure I was kept comfortable during the surgery and throughout the recovery.

Additionally, prior to the surgery, I had spent time contemplating what pain really was. I learned to rate it from 1-10 and appreciate the different forms, reactions and durations of pain. Thus, when I felt any pain, I often got lost in my thoughts as I contemplated which form of pain I had, measuring and analyzing the intensity. In most cases, it was gone before I could fully process it.

Should one expect this experience to be completely pain-free? Of course not. Any person who even considers kidney donation understands there is an element of personal sacrifice – giving of oneself for the sake of others.

However, this paradigm is not exclusive to kidney donation. Each and every living being that walks the earth is a product and symbol of a selfless sacrifice. When a mother voluntarily allows herself to endure 9 months of discomfort, followed by the incredible pain of childbirth, she models for us the extent one goes to give life. It is no surprise, therefore, that the Hebrew word for compassion (*rechem*), is the same word for womb, as it suggests that giving life is the ultimate in compassion and selflessness. While nobody *wants* to experience pain, I felt it was a small price to pay in contrast to what I would ultimately be giving.

Chapter 6.
Recovering in the Hospital

66. What should I expect when I wake up?

The first thing I was told to expect after surgery was to feel tired and sleepy. This was spot on. When I first woke up, I was extremely drowsy, as the anesthesia lingers in the body even after the surgery is over. Since it takes time for the full effects to completely wear off, I was encouraged to rest and sleep, while my body recovered.

Although I was concerned I would be in terrible pain when I woke up from surgery, I actually had the opposite experience. Surprisingly, I felt no pain at all. In fact, in the recovery room when I opened my eyes, I was unsure of whether or not I even had the surgery. After all, I was feeling calm and comfortable, as if I just woke up from a nice afternoon nap! Lying cozy in bed under many layers of warm blankets, I remember running my hand down my stomach and even pressing on my abdomen to see if it hurt. I just could not believe the surgery was over. I was certainly able to detect the feeling of pressure as I foolishly pressed on my abdomen, but I knew the pain medications were doing their job perfectly.

Additionally, I was given a *beloved* morphine button which I was able to press when I felt any pain. Within seconds, the morphine administered through the IV kicked in and helped stop any pain. Additionally, during that first day on morphine, it built up in my system and continued to maintain my comfort throughout the rest of the night and into the following morning, even when I was not actively pressing the button.

67. Will my family be able to come to the recovery room?

While I was resting comfortably in the post-op recovery room, the surgeon called my wife who was sitting in the waiting room to update her and allowed her to visit me. As a general rule, they tend not bring more than one or two people to visit patients in the recovery room at any given time. Having my wife at my side was not only comforting on an emotional level, but she was very helpful to me practically as well while I rested in my loopy, dream-like semi-consciousness.

After having seen my share of funny viral videos of cruel, but well-intentioned family members who recorded their loved ones after surgery as they acted silly or incoherent, my wife and I had made a pact. She agreed in advance that nothing I said in my drug-induced state "could or would be used against me." There was, however, one cute story that stands out, which she and I still joke about.

Because my lips were very dry, my wife was kind enough to stand at my side and moisten them with a swab dipped in cool water. It may seem like a small thing, but it really helped make me feel so much more comfortable. With my eyes closed, I drifted in and out of sleep, and every few minutes I would pucker my lips outward as a sign they were again feeling dry. On cue, my wife was kind enough to swab them with cool water. However, one time, while lying there half asleep, I pushed my lips out, but nothing. I did it again and again, but no response. I opened one eye and realized my wife had stepped aside to speak to one of the nurses, just standing a few feet away. In my drug-induced, dream-like rationale, I thought to myself, "hmmm, if only I had a bell I could swing in the air, it would be the perfect way to call her over, without having to summon the energy to actually call out for her."

Realizing at the moment that despite all of my thorough preparation, I had failed to think about bringing a bell, I came up with an alternative in what seemed like a good idea at the time. I figured that I could just use my hand as a bell. Therefore, I raised my arm over the side of the bed and began swinging my hand back and forth. After a few moments, she looked curiously across the room and noticed that I was waving my wrist in the air. She asked if I was OK and what I was doing. I just responded by waving my hand again and declaring, "ding-a-ling a-ling, ding-a-ling a-ling" and then puckering my lips."

She burst out laughing at my ingenuity, at which point I joined in amusement, as it quickly occurred to me that my hand was not in fact a bell. Thank God she was a good sport and had a great sense of humor, and was able to appreciate the medication was certainly doing its job. To this day, we still joke when trying to get each other's attention, by waving a wrist in the air and calling out, "ding-a-ling a-ling."

68. Will there be any nausea after the surgery?

As anesthesia has been known to sometimes cause an upset stomach, part of the standard medication regimen includes something to prevent nausea.

Even though it may seem trite, like many people, I hate feeling nauseous, and even more, I despise the sickness which may follow. On a good day nobody enjoys vomiting, however, following abdominal surgery, I was concerned about the pain it would cause if I were to get sick. Because of my own added fears, I was instructed by the transplant coordinator to raise my concern ahead of time with the anesthesiologist, who was very receptive and understanding. I explained that I have a sensitive stomach and really did not want to have any problems. The doctors, therefore, provided me with the standard anti-nausea medications, as well as something extra. I was really releived that throughout the surgery and recovery process, I never felt sick and had no problems with nausea or vomiting. The nurses were also instructed to continue to deliver anti-nausea medications on the following day, as well as on an as-needed basis, should I feel any nausea. There were a few moments on the day following surgery when my stomach was feeling a little bit unsettled. Not wanting to take any chances, I asked the nurse, who gladly provided me with an extra dose, which helped immediately settle my stomach and prevent any further discomfort.

This experience further highlights the importance of preparation. By discussing this particular concern in advance, additional steps were then able to be taken in order to prevent any problems.

69. How soon before I will be able to get out of bed?

I was quite surprised when I learned early on in the process, that the hospital will get patients out of bed on the day following surgery. The basic rule is the more a patient walks around, the quicker they will diffuse the lingering anesthesia and the effects of surgery from their body and jump start a faster recovery process.

The practicality of getting out of bed, however, is somewhat of a double-edged sword. On one hand, the body still has the lingering effects of anesthesia, which means that the patient will be drowsy and fatigued. On the other hand, the patient has a good amount of morphine built up in their system, which prevents them from feeling too much discomfort. For me, this combination meant that mentally I was ready to jump right out of bed, but physically, I barely had the energy to swing my tired legs off the side of the bed.

Thus, within 24 hours of surgery, with lots of patience and encouragement from nurses, I was helped to my feet. Being a typical guy, I took great pride in each step I took, slowly shuffling across the room to sit in a chair. Despite my moans and groans, with a room full of people cheering me on, I felt like an Olympic athlete crossing the finish line.

However, before I had the opportunity to celebrate too much, my inflated ego was quickly brought back down to earth. As I sat in the chair, ready to celebrate my heroic five steps, the door to my room began to open. I looked up to see who it was. Yet, instead of seeing a person, I observed a hand, holding on to an IV pole, as it was slowly being wheeled into the room. To my utter disbelief, tracing behind the pole was Ronit, as she slowly shuffled her way into my room, trying to hide any discomfort behind a huge smile on her face.

Needless to say, I was extremely humbled by her efforts, as she was also a mere 24 hours post-surgery. I looked up and asked, "Ronit, what are you doing here, why aren't you in bed?"

She smiled and shrugged her shoulders as she answered me with two simple Hebrew words, *Bikkur Cholim* – "visiting the sick."

There I was, somewhat shamefully celebrating my few steps to the chair, while Ronit had managed to walk from her room, down the hall, across a corridor and into my room. For me, that was both humbling and inspiring!

My eyes began to well up with tears as I realized the heroic efforts she exerted to perform her own act of kindness. All along, I viewed her as the one who was not well, but in this moment, she was so filled with gratitude and compassion that she felt compelled to check on my recovery. I could not have been more moved by her gesture. Having seen Ronit in action so soon after the surgery, really reinforced for me just how precious that little five-ounce gift was to her.

From a medical perspective, it is not uncommon for the kidney recipient to demonstrate a quicker bounce-back than the donor. Because the recipient's body has grown accustomed to functioning with little to no kidney function prior to transplant, every day is filled with physical fatigue and a mental haze. As soon as one receives the new kidney, it is as if a cloud has been lifted and the body begins to operate at a capacity that it may not have met in years. In fact, the new kidney is so powerful in the recipient's body, that even following open abdominal surgery and with the lingering effects of anesthesia, the recipient still feels a dramatic improvement! It is for this reason as well, that the recipient often demonstrates a very meaningful resilience as they begin the first day of their "new" lives.

In contrast, the donor, who may otherwise have been in excellent health prior to surgery, is now beginning a new reality post-surgery. This is when the remaining kidney actually grows in size and learns to jump into overdrive to begin the process of taking on the workload of two kidneys, something it is perfectly capable of doing. Due to this shift, it is normal for the donor to initially report feeling more tired, while the recipient feels more energized.

70. What should I expect during the first night in the hospital?

With the help of the morphine keeping me comfortable, and the urinary catheter allowing me to rest without running to the bathroom, I was surprised at how comfortable I was on the night after surgery. My mother was kind enough to stay with me during the first night, as she camped out in a chair next to my bed. Between drifting in and out of sleep, we talked, joked and watched TV and before long the sun came up.

There is a long-standing joke known by anyone who has ever slept in a hospital. It is the only place where someone will wake you up in the middle of the night just to give you a sleeping pill!

While this was not my exact experience, one should be prepared for nurses checking-in throughout the night. Although it may seem frustrating for some who are trying to sleep, I found it to be reassuring, knowing the medical team was constantly keeping an eye on me - even if it meant waking me up to check my vital signs and see how I was feeling.

71. How can I expedite the recovery process?

Walking is the single best thing a patient can do after surgery. Despite the boredom of walking laps around a hospital corridor, walking helps the body shake the effects of surgery. One may not consciously be aware of it, but the heart, lungs, digestive track and other organs feel the impact of anesthesia and walking helps them recover. Following surgery, I was given what looked like a toddler's toy. In fact, it was an Incentive Spirometer, which is a clear plastic device with a ball inside and a tube coming out of it. When a patient inhales on the tube, the ball rises. It is designed to help keep the patient's lungs clear by encouraging deep breathing. Without this little device, a patient may be slower to recover and may face increased risk of breathing complications, such as pneumonia.

I remember being shown this device before surgery and with a tiny bit of effort inhaled on the tube, sending the ball directly to the top. After surgery, I attempted to do the same thing expecting similar results. However, despite trying my hardest, I was only able to raise the ball to hover midway up the device. I was astonished by how challenging it was. After all, I thought my lungs felt great and did not notice any limitation on my breathing following surgery.

It was at this point I realized the importance of rehabilitating all parts of the body. As per the doctor's instructions, I practiced a few times each hour and slowly improved my score. By the time I left the hospital, I was able to quickly raise the ball to the top of the device and proudly keep it in place. Seeing the measurable progress unfold before my eyes was an encouraging sign of how quickly the body heals with each passing hour and each passing day.

72. How is my pain managed during my recovery?

Following surgery my pain was well managed with a morphine button as well as oral narcotics. Honestly, I felt great! The goal for the next few days was to quickly move away from the morphine and graduate to only using the oral narcotics as needed, followed next by Tylenol (with a codeine option to be used if I needed help sleeping at night).

The fact that the nurses would have to wake me up on the first night to check on me, was a testament to just how comfortable and pain-free I was feeling. However, this led to somewhat of a misstep. Due to the fact that I was feeling *so* good, when asked if I was ready to move to oral narcotic medication, I declined. After all, I did not want to take more medicine than I needed. I was quite impressed with my ability to rest so comfortably the entire first night without taking anything but Tylenol. I naively assumed I was out of the woods and well on my way to a quick recovery. I later learned that my comfort during the night was due to the morphine and anesthesia which lingered in my body.

What I soon confronted was the fact that the morphine wore off, and Tylenol was not a strong enough solution. When I started noticing some discomfort, I discussed it with my nurse. She reminded me there was no need to be a martyr, especially on the first day after surgery! That is when I realized that I had jumped the gun with regard to weaning myself from the pain medications, which were necessary in supporting me through the recovery. I then resumed oral narcotics, per the doctor's instructions, and remained on them while I was in the hospital and during the first day or two after returning home.

One additional source of discomfort patients may experience is shoulder pain - a common side-effect of laparoscopic surgery. This is because during a laparoscopic surgery, the abdomen is inflated with air to help surgeons better see what they are doing. Even though the air is let out as the transplant is completed, the diaphragm can become irritated in the process and the excess air bubbles may temporarily linger in the body. Thus, it may take a day or two for them to become fully absorbed and escape the body.

I remember this distinct discomfort during my second night at the hospital. While it was not painful per se, the feeling was not a comfortable one. It was comparable to having eaten way too much for dinner and then following it with a large carbonated beverage. The more I would sit up and walk around, the more the tiny air bubbles would rise up and collect beneath my skin causing discomfort. As I would run my hand along the surface of my shoulders and chest, I could actually feel the bubbles dissipating and disappearing. With that, the feeling of discomfort disappeared as well.

The main lesson I learned regarding pain management was exactly as my nurse had said - don't be a martyr. If a patient ever feels any pain, they should bring it up with their nurse so that it can be properly addressed. A pain management plan is carefully put in place to help donors and there is no reason for any patient to try and be a hero, as it will not accelerate the recovery process. Instead, sit back, follow the plan and enjoy the trip.

73. What type of food will I be allowed to eat in the hospital?

While there are no specific restrictions to what a person can or cannot eat in the hospital, many patients have a small appetite following surgery. It is important for patients to find foods that are not only appealing, but also light and easily digestible. In addition to having a "sleepy digestive tract" after surgery, it is common for people on morphine and narcotic pain medication to experience some constipation. With that in mind, eating the right foods can make life simpler.

To prevent additional discomfort, patients are given stool softeners and laxatives (or what my nurse lovingly phrased as, "the mushers and the pushers") to aid in worry-free digestion. By eating foods that are high in fiber and drinking lots of fluids, a patient can reduce the strains of what could otherwise be a more challenging bowel movement. Ultimately, the less stress the patient puts on their abdominal muscles and digestive system, the more comfortable they will be.

74. While I recover, how am I monitored?

By watching a patient's basic vital signs, such as blood pressure and body temperature, the doctors can be extra vigilant in identifying any additional stress on the body - such as complications or signs of infection. In the event something seems out of the ordinary, the medical team can be quick to react with antibiotics or pain medication as needed.

Additionally, doctors will be measuring urine output, which is a great sign the remaining kidney is functioning as expected. Not only will they be assessing the quantity of urine, but looking at the quality of it as well. This includes measuring the color, protein content, electrolytes and creatinine (which indicates the level of kidney function).

75. How long must I stay in the hospital?

While a hospital stay for kidney donation can range from 1-7 days, the average stay for a laparoscopic procedure is only 2 days! While a patient will be allowed to stay in the hospital as long as medically necessary, assuming everything is going according to plan, they will be assessed to go home on the day after surgery. In my case, I went to the hospital on Monday morning for the surgery and on Tuesday afternoon was I able to go home. However, patients are offered an additional "flex day," giving them the option to stay a third day, should they choose to do so.

In the medical community, the benefits of this additional day are debated. Some doctors feel that a patient who is stable and comfortable can just as easily recover at home. Thus, keeping them in the hospital (which is generally full of sick people), may increase the risk of exposing them to germs they did carry when they first came to the hospital. This school of thought would prefer that patients who are ready to leave do so as soon as possible.

The other side of the debate argues that a patient may do better while under direct medical care of doctors and nurses, and thus spending the extra day in the hospital would prove to be beneficial.

When I entered the hospital, I did so with an open mind. I figured if I was feeling well enough to leave on day two, I would be discharged. However, if I felt I needed the extra day, I would be open to taking it. When the time came to make the decision, I felt as if I could go either way. However, as I found myself growing far stronger with each passing hour of each day, I decided to remain in the comforts of the hospital for an additional night, and was discharged in the late morning of day three. In hindsight, I can confirm it was the right decision for me. Having direct access to my medical team to answer questions, plus having a bed which could sit up or recline with the press of a button made life that much easier, and brought me a touch more comfort as I began the transition from hospital to normal life.

Chapter 7.
Recovering at Home

76. What is the recovery like at home?

After being discharged, I sat in a wheelchair and was pushed to the hospital lobby. My wife brought the car around and the nurses patiently helped me climb in. When we arrived home, I stepped out of the car and took a moment to appreciate the sunshine and fresh air. As I slowly walked up the stairs and into the house, I prepared my mind for what would begin the next stage of my journey, the home-recovery.

I was ready to climb into bed and continue to enjoy my sweet rest, when my blissful bubble was quickly burst. As my wife helped me through the door, she looked at me with a smile and lovingly, but firmly said, "now go take a shower and get into bed." I thought she was crazy. I just got out of the hospital and wanted to rest, not shower. Yet, she would not take no for an answer. She reminded me it was time to start feeling like a human being again, not a patient. Her advice was right on the money.

My wife started the shower and set up everything I would need, and then closed the door behind her.

Very slowly and carefully, I began a new process. This was the first time since I entered the hospital I would have some quiet, all by myself. It was an opportunity for me to wash away the "patient" and begin to feel like "Ari."

Surprisingly, more than just being a physical experience, I found the shower to be an emotionally and psychologically profound one. It was during that time when the enormity of my kidney donation really began to sink in. I was able to explore and embrace the small, but meaningful scars which I would carry with me for life. I was introduced to the permanent reminders of just how special this experience had been for me, and more importantly, for Ronit and her family.

I stepped out of the shower a different person. Feeling not only clean and refreshed, but more human, I was ready to begin my own future, starting with the next stage of my recovery.

I entered a new temporary reality. It was one of spending the next few days focused on getting back on my feet. This involved two basic ingredients: resting and walking. When the weather was nice, I went outside for a walk. Initially, it was just to the end of the driveway and back. The following day it was to the end of the street. By Friday, with my fast-paced music playing, I was very slowly but surely walking several laps around the block. When the weather was less cooperative, I would simply walk laps around the house just to continue my recovery and regain my strength.

In between meals and walking, I rested and relaxed, watched some TV, and occasionally took a nap when needed. To keep my days and nights separate, I tried to avoid staying in bed, unless it was nighttime. Rotating between different couches and chairs kept me out of bed and allowed me to relax while also moving and having a change of scenery. I also pushed myself each morning to change from my "sleeping" sweat pants into my "daytime" ones. Although there was little difference between my two wardrobes, symbolically, it helped me feel more human during the day, rather than living in my pajamas for a week. The recovery process was just as much psychological as it was physical, and these small strategies made a significant difference.

77. Will I be in pain?

There were only two circumstances at home, when I really felt any serious pain. Ironically, the first was due to pure laughter. You see, many well-intentioned people wished to add some color to my life by visiting me at home as I recuperated. I soon noticed, that as a means of lightening the mood, they were inclined to joke around and try to make me laugh. Ouch!! As crazy as it sounds, laughter was probably the most painful part of the entire process. It was only after I found myself laughing so hard, that I realized how much the contraction of abdominal muscles can hurt following surgery.

Upon realizing the complete absurdity and irony of how feeling happy could hurt so much, only made me laugh harder! Ultimately, I found myself laughing and crying at the same time, in what was a truly hysterical moment. I don't quite recall what specific expletives I used to get my friends to stop cracking jokes, but I'm sure they were not for the faint of heart. After a few moments, I left the room to catch my breath and returned once I had regained my composure and given my abdominal muscles a respite from laughter. I also found it helpful to hold a pillow against my stomach, to ease the pain that laughter brought. Despite the discomfort I experienced at the time, I still look back at those funny moments and once again laugh - now without any pain.

The second circumstance in which I felt abdominal discomfort was when switching positions from lying down to sitting up and vice versa. Most people do not realize just how much they depend on their core stomach muscles to accomplish something as simple as getting out of bed. At first, I tried to just pull myself up, which was not pleasant. After a day or two I figured out the trick of the trade. The best way to get out of bed was to slowly roll onto my side and gently ease myself up. Here too, holding a pillow against my stomach gave me a little extra strength and comfort, as I engaged the recovering muscles. Initially, it was most helpful to have another person there to help me roll and sit up, until I learned to perfect the maneuver and stick the landing.

I also found it helpful during those first few days to have many extra pillows on my bed, so I would not have to lay completely flat and engage those core stomach muscles more than necessary. Resting in somewhat of a sitting or inclined position gave me more flexibility to get up with less discomfort. Additionally, I took great comfort in having a hot water bottle I could place on my abdomen whenever the muscles felt sore. It was a small, but soothing thing, which really made a big difference in keeping me more comfortable. Within about a week these concerns were mostly gone, as I was getting stronger and faster at doing these simple tasks.

78. What medications will I take at home?

When I was discharged from the hospital, I was sent home with medications as well as additional prescriptions to use in the event they were necessary. Part of my discharge instructions included the use of narcotics to help with pain management. However, I only found them necessary to use for the two days at home. After all, using the heavier medications made me feel tired and loopy, a feeling which I did not particularly enjoy, nor did they allow me to go for the necessary walks which would expedite my recovery.

Therefore, when I realized I could cope without narcotics, I switched to using Tylenol to manage any discomfort. For the first two nights, I opted for the Tylenol with codeine, which helped me fall into a good deep sleep. After that, I only used regular Tylenol as needed, and found I was generally very comfortable. I continued to take the stool softeners, which helped aid in the digestion process, reducing the need for straining core abdominal muscles. Overall, managing the pain was an extremely comfortable experience - even more so with the right preparation, tools and support.

79. Are there any other short-term risks I should be worried about?

As with any surgical procedure, patients are universally told to look out for signs of infection — development of a fever, or any unusual redness around the incision sites. Additionally, doctors want to make sure that the remaining kidney is functioning as it should, and, therefore, if the donor notices anything unusual, he or she should contact the hospital. However, for most people, myself included, the recovery process was smooth and uneventful, and without complications.

As questions or concerns arose during my first few days home, I found it helpful to have the transplant coordinator's phone number programmed into my phone, so I had immediate access to the answers I was looking for. Sometimes, just having that little bit of additional reassurance goes a long way in offering extra peace of mind. I was reminded of the many wonderful people I had in my corner, who were supporting me during this incredible journey.

80. At what point do I go from being a patient to feeling like myself again?

There is a fine balance every patient should strive for. On one hand, it is important to initially embrace the patient mentality. It is this mindset allows one to take it slow, enjoy the help and support of those around them, and do so without pushing oneself too much, or too quickly.

On the other hand, it is important at the right time to break free from the patient mentality and begin thinking and acting like a regular healthy person.

From a physical standpoint, this is done in phases as a patient slowly regains his or her strength and energy. Psychologically, however, the sooner one can get into the frame of mind of, "I'm better," the more likely one is to shed the sluggishness that may come with the recovery process.

Another example of this was during the first week of recovery when I found it tiring to have long conversations. It did not mean I was incapable of doing work, for I felt great mentally - I just could not yet return to my normal physical demands. Therefore, I started slowly by sitting comfortably with a laptop, sending emails and keeping up with work and correspondence. This allowed me to make the transition from feeling like a patient, to feeling fully productive again. It was helpful to be in touch with both my physical and mental abilities. Just because I felt physically tired did not mean that my mind was not sharp or capable of being productive.

81. Are there any additional restrictions following surgery?

To keep the incision site dry, clean and free from bacteria buildup, one should not soak in a tub or swim in a pool for the first few weeks. Following a shower, it is important to pat dry the bandages and surgical areas, so bacteria does not breed in the moist areas, which could lead to an increased chance of infection.

82. How should I expect to feel emotionally?

Much of the literature regarding the emotional state of a kidney donor following surgery is compared to that of a woman following childbirth. Just as there may be pain and discomfort associated with bringing a child into this world, it is nevertheless, quickly justified by the magnitude of the accomplishment. After all, how can one express the joy that accompanies giving life, or the lengths to which one would go in order to do so?

I recall feeling a sense of euphoric pride and deep inner fulfillment – a feeling that still stays with me even years later! Yet, in some cases of kidney donation, much like childbirth, there are reports of what some describe akin to post-partum depression.

When a woman experiences the journey of pregnancy, there is something miraculous about it. She walks around feeling special, knowing there is a higher purpose to her existence, as she is constantly nurturing and sustaining life within her own body.

However, once the child is born, even though, she can finally celebrate the feelings of joy associated with seeing, holding and embracing the baby, she may feel a wave of sadness for no longer having that same internal sense of purpose. The post-partum blues are often described as a mourning period for a mother losing the potential to sustain another life within her own body.

The same phenomenon can take place with kidney donors. There are some patients, who after spending months preparing themselves and nurturing the kidney within them to be transferred to another person, experience a sadness once it is all over. While there is immeasurable joy in the knowledge of having saved a human life, some people feel an emotional void, knowing the donation is complete, and the life-saving gift that grew within them is no longer a part of them.

It is helpful for kidney donors to be mindful of these emotions and to discuss them openly with the transplant coordinator, particularly if a person has a history of depression or mood disorders. In most cases, post-donation blues pass quickly. However, in the event that the feelings linger, or a donor experiences depression, it should be quickly and unabashedly addressed, so it may be treated with therapy and readily available medications.

Personally, I did not experience any post-donation sadness. Rather, like most donors, I carry the joys of the experience with me every day of my life.

83. Does kidney donation affect physical intimacy?

Through my research, I learned that men and women have different concerns for how kidney donation might impact their sex life, and the question is quite common. Yet, like all of my researched questions, I wanted to ask a doctor myself. However, it was the type of question I simply could not seem to find the right time to ask.

When the question finally popped into my head, my wife and I were in the middle of a consultation with a young medical intern. She was new to the field and was heavily focused on explaining renal function and kidney transplantation, until I abruptly changed the topic to ask this question.

Although the doctor was a professional, she was caught off guard and immediately turned beet red. She began getting all flustered as she stammered, struggling to form a coherent clinical answer. My wife and I both looked at each other and we all just broke out laughing. After a few moments of laughter, awkward smiles, a deep breath and brief reset, she answered the question, and clarified that kidney donation does not impact one's sex life. The only limitation to be mindful is during the initial recovery period, when one should not strain the muscles which are recuperating.

84. When can I return to the gym?

To best protect the patient during the first week or two of recovery, doctors instruct patients not to carry or lift anything more than 10-15 pounds in weight, so as not to stress the core abdominal muscles, which could lead to increased possibility of developing a hernia. After that point, with each passing week, one may slowly increase their weight load.

Thus, even though I began to gradually exercise, my first few weeks were limited to walking, and eventually some slow jogging and I avoided any weight-lifting or abdominal exercises. After I cleared the first month and with doctor's approval, I began to steadily incorporate some light weightlifting and more strenuous exercises, but always took great care to cautiously listen to my body, so as not to push myself too far, too fast.

85. When can I return to work?

For most people the one-week mark is an important milestone. In my case, after the first week, I felt about 65% back to myself again. With each passing day I felt exponentially stronger. After week two, I was operating at about 80% capacity - at which point, I even had a business trip, and had no problem navigating the airport or flights. I only had to be mindful of restricting the weight of my carry-on bag not to exceed 10-15 lbs. Over the course of the following few weeks, I gradually returned to about 95% of my full strength and then continued to close the gap until I was back to 100%. Even during the first few months when I was generally feeling back to myself, from time to time, I would get a reminder to slow down, as I would feel slightly tired or fatigued. Those little experiences were brief, but nevertheless important cues for me to listen to my body and allow myself to fully recover.

Thus, for a person who works a desk job, returning to work within 2 weeks should be a perfectly reasonable goal. Obviously, for someone who works a physical or manual labor job, it is important to allow at least 4-6 weeks before returning to any form of lifting and to get a doctor's clearance before returning to work.

86. Can I drive right away?

While a kidney donor may feel perfectly capable of driving after surgery, it is advised to wait at least a few weeks and as many as six-weeks. The reason for this is twofold. Firstly, patients must be careful not to drive while still taking pain medications which can cause drowsiness or delayed reactions and put them, or others, in harm's way.

Furthermore, even if a patient is no longer taking pain medication, driving a car requires the ability to slam on the brakes if necessary. A patient following surgery, will be slower to react, and will be more careful to favor their "injury" by not making any sudden moves which could hurt them. As a result, the discharge notes from the hospital will instruct patients specifically to avoid driving a car, as they may not have the full ability to react as quickly as necessary to drive safely.

87. What kind of support system will I need?

The kidney donation process is not something that one can go through on their own. While the testing, research, and preparation may seem like a personal journey, it culminates in an experience that requires the help and support of others. For me, it did not only include having someone who can stay with me overnight in the hospital, drive me around after surgery, help bring me meals, or get in and out of bed, but rather, having the emotional and moral support was crucial. While there may be people in every donor's life who disagree with the decision to donate, it will be particularly helpful in the recovery process to be surrounded by a handful of amazing and supportive people. The more the donor is supported, the better off he or she will recover and thrive.

For instance, a mom who is donating a kidney needs the peace of mind that someone can help watch her children; lift the laundry; or drive carpool while she is recuperating. Certainly, during the first two weeks after surgery a household cannot operate under the premise of "business as usual." Having friends and family available to help lend a hand will go a very long way.

Such help, should not be committed in theory, but in very concrete terms. The daily responsibilities that must be tended to in life, should be delegated to specific people who can best carry them out. As there may be a surge of support during the first several days after surgery, it would be helpful to come up with a list or a rotation of people who are available to continue helping after things quiet down but while additional assistance is still needed.

I cannot recall the number of times in my career I have seen kind-hearted people jump at the opportunity to offer support to others in need. However, at the time when the help is actually needed, there is nobody to be found. When someone is facing a hardship, whether being hospitalized; losing a relative; going through a divorce; or, suffering an illness, you can inevitably hear the words, "please let me know if you need anything." While the offer is sincere, it is seldom delivered upon. This is because people in crisis do not need "anything," they need something specific. If I had a dollar for every casserole that I have seen delivered to people in crisis, I'd be set for life. Meals are often the go-to option for delivering good thoughts, love, and acts of kindness, but there are often many other practical ways to take care of people in need.

As one might expect, kidney donors tend to be very giving people. As such, they are often less inclined to accept help, and may be particularly reluctant to ask for it from others. This is when it is most important to remember that kidney donation is a team effort. Just as in football, only one person scores the touchdown, but it is the result of the entire team coordinating the pass and the blocking. So too, with kidney donation, only one person actually donates the kidney, but the entire team plays a role in helping to make it happen. The more thought that goes into preparing, planning and coordinating the details in advance, the more smooth the overall process will be.

Chapter 8.
The Rest of My Life

88.   Will I have to take medications for the rest of my life?

No, this is actually a common misconception. The donor does not have to take any life-long medications as a result of the donation. However, the recipient does. These are commonly known as anti-rejection medications. The recipient's immune system recognizes the new kidney as being a foreign object in the body, and the natural reaction is to fight it. Therefore, the anti-rejection medication suppresses the recipient's immune system to help ensure their body accepts the new kidney. The more closely matched the donor and recipient are, the fewer medications will be required.

I recall the moment I first realized the importance of recipients taking their daily anti-rejection medications. It was when I first met Ronit and she could not stop thanking me profusely. While we were both teary-eyed and smiling from ear to ear, she leaned over and said, "I want you to know that I promise you that I will take my medications every single day."

At first, I thought that it was a rather strange comment to make when you meet a stranger for the first time. However, after a moment, it sunk in and I realized what she was truly saying. Unfortunately, there are recipients who are blessed to receive the gift of life from someone who generously gives them a kidney, but they fail to take it seriously. As a result, they miss a few days here and there of their anti-rejection medications, and eventually, the donated kidney begins to fail. Soon after, they are put back on dialysis and once again begin the process of awaiting a new kidney. All the while, that organ could have gone to someone else who would have cared for it properly.

What Ronit was telling me was just how much she valued the gift I was giving her, and how she would never take it for granted. Her commitment to taking the daily medications was Ronit's way of expressing her partnership with me and assuring me that my sacrifice would be met by her own level of devotion to the process. Needless to say, once I fully understood what she meant, it helped me appreciate what an amazing new home Ronit would give my kidney.

89. Do I have to drink extra water every day?

A kidney donor is not required to drink more water than anyone else. However, the reality is that most people tend not to drink the minimum suggested amount of water per day. Therefore, to best care for their remaining kidney, donors should be mindful each day to drink ample water and stay hydrated. This is a great way to keep the kidney safe and healthy. Donors who tend to be outdoors during the hot summer months, or living in warmer climates, should be sure to keep extra water on hand.

90. Are there any long-term risks to be concerned about?

The primary concerns for donors are similar to those of the general population. Heart disease and high blood pressure are among the biggest threats today for the general population. Kidney donors, however, will have an increased chance of high blood pressure and should maintain a reasonably healthy diet and include some exercise in their weekly routine. This will help ensure their blood pressure continue at a normal and healthy level.

It is still important, however, for donors to be mindful of their blood pressure. Like many donors, I keep a digital blood-pressure cuff in my night stand and check my numbers every few months just to ensure everything looks good. Each year, at my annual physical, the doctor checks my blood pressure and urine to ensure my heart and kidney are both functioning well. In the event one develops high blood pressure, just like other adults in the general population, the doctor will likely prescribe a daily oral medication to keep their numbers in check and reduce any additional strain on the heart.

In addition to living a lifestyle of healthy diet and exercise, drinking water will keep the kidney well-hydrated, as well as contribute to a healthier blood pressure. I have grown accustomed to keeping a bottle of water next to my bed and taking a quick drink when I go to sleep and when I wake up. I have found that doing so has helped increase my energy level as I start my day, to the extent that I now feel even better in the morning than I did before I donated my kidney.

91. Will I be able to still drink alcohol or coffee?

Yes, a kidney donor can drink alcohol and coffee without any problem. This is something I have since personally tested and proven. However, like all things in life, moderation is always the smart practice, especially for a kidney donor who now embarks upon life with a heightened appreciation for maintaining his or her health.

Keep in mind that alcohol and coffee tend to dehydrate the body, and should not serve as a replacement for drinking water. Thus, if one drinks several cups of coffee in the morning, or has a few beers at night, it should be balanced with drinking ample water.

92. Are there any medical limitations or changes to my life?

Following kidney donation and for the rest of my life, doctors instructed me to avoid using ibuprofen, such as Motrin and Advil. This category of medications, also known as NSAIDs (non-steroidal anti-inflammatory drugs) are avoided because, as anti-inflammatory medications, they can impact blood flow, which has the potential to cause damage to one's kidney. While they can be helpful to reduce pain, and are often used to reduce inflammation, such as for those with arthritis, NSAID's come with many added health risks to the stomach, kidneys, liver and heart.

Therefore, kidney donors should instead rely on using Tylenol or other Acetaminophen products, which are the most commonly used over-the-counter pain medications for reducing fevers, headaches, aches and pains. Although some doctors occasionally permit ibuprofen in small quantities and doses, others prefer that kidney donors avoid it altogether. As with all medical questions, each person should carefully consult their own doctor.

93. Can I still get pregnant?

Okay, this was not exactly a question I asked before deciding to donate a kidney. Yet, since it is a very important question many women ask, I felt it should be addressed within this book.

The answer is, yes! All the literature I have seen suggests pregnancy following kidney donation is safe. One should, however, postpone pregnancy at least 3-6 months following kidney donation to allow ample time for the body to heal.

Because in some cases, pregnancy may increase blood pressure, one should discuss this, and all other pregnancy-related questions with their doctor in advance. There are some female donors who have chosen to wait a few extra years before donating a kidney, so they could first have children and alleviate any of their concerns regarding pregnancy following donation. Then, after completing their child-bearing years, they can once again continue to give life through kidney donation!

94. What kind of follow-up care do I need after the donation?

After being discharged from the hospital, I was asked to return one week later, and then again within the month. This was to ensure the incisions were healing properly and my kidney was functioning at capacity. After the first month, most programs will check on donors again within six months, a year, or even annually. The ultimate goal, however, is to graduate to using one's primary care physician for all routine checkups.

Donors should make sure their hospital and regular physician are in contact with one another so any important information or findings can be easily shared and discussed. As long as one is seeing their doctor annually, there is no need for any additional follow-up care specific to kidney donation.

95. Are there any limitations for my "athletic life?"

My wife chuckled when I so much as pondered this question. Knowing I am hardly the athletic type she thought it was funny I was concerned about my future as a professional athlete. The nature of the question was more related to knowing about any potential physical limitations, than it was my ability to be a first-draft pick in professional sports.

While it may not relate to my lifestyle, the short answer to this question is yes, there can be limitations to a kidney donor's athletic future. However, having one kidney does not inherently limit a person's physical ability. The limitations are self-imposed to protect the remaining kidney from activities that may cause injury.

The rule is, any sport or activity that can potentially damage the kidney should be avoided. For instance, someone who is preparing to fight in the Ultimate Fighting Champion; is engaged in mixed-martial arts; or, plays tackle football, should consider the serious risks of such activities on the remaining kidney. Additionally, if one is currently in the military, or planning to join, he or she should first explore whether having one kidney could impact his or her ability to serve in various capacities.

Personally, since I did not have any significant athletic aspirations, I was not concerned about such limitations. The majority of my physical activities include jogging and some weight training, which contribute to my health, and do not run the risk of causing any damage to my kidney.

Recently, I undertook the challenge of training for a half-marathon, and even with one kidney, impressed myself with the pace and stamina that I maintained. After kidney donation, one should continue to enjoy an active lifestyle, provided that they are not engaging in any particularly dangerous activities.

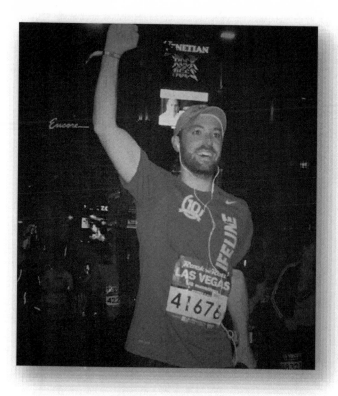

Dare I say, that because I live with a heightened awareness to maintain my health, I am now living a far healthier lifestyle than I was prior to my kidney donation. My mindfulness about diet and exercise have helped me maintain a way of life that has increased my energy level and productivity. Thus, even with only one kidney, I enjoy a healthier lifestyle than many of my "two-kidney" contemporaries.

96. Will I have trouble obtaining health insurance after donating a kidney?

Before delving too far into the exploration process, I called my insurance company to make sure I would not have any problems obtaining health insurance in the future. Because this was a voluntary procedure, I was concerned that it might impact my ability to obtain coverage.

While I was assured I was fully covered before, during and after the procedure, I was still concerned about what might happen to my coverage long into the future. However, with the introduction of the Affordable Care Act, insurance companies can no longer deny coverage based on preexisting conditions.

This new reality is another measure which helps further protect kidney donors. Additionally, there is new legislation being presented, which specifically aims to establish new policies that provide additional protection to kidney donors and promote healthy, safe and ethical kidney donation.

97. Will I have trouble obtaining life insurance?

Many people are uncomfortable discussing life insurance (which should more aptly be named death insurance). However, as I was proceeding through the kidney donation exploration, my wife and I had a very blunt conversation. Our goal throughout the process was to leave no stone unturned and examine every possibility and contingency. Since preparation was our motto, it included confirming that both my life and disability insurance policies would provide the coverage we needed in the unlikely event something went wrong during the surgery. This might seem morose to some people, but we felt it necessary to be as thorough as possible and to take every step toward ensuring our financial protection. With one simple phone call to our insurance agent, we were given peace of mind as my coverage would not change, nor would my rates increase as a result of the donation.

As there are countless insurance companies and agencies, it is strongly advised for potential donors to carefully look into their current and potential future insurance options. While most donors have not had difficulty obtaining or maintaining their insurance, there have been some reports of people who have either been denied, or charged higher rates due to their donation. In many cases, one can work with their transplant hospital to help educate the insurance company on the research which verifies the health of kidney donors as the same or better than the general population.

Chapter 9.
Conclusion

98. Doesn't it make sense to keep my second kidney just in case?

With great humility, I realized throughout this process that nobody can see the future or know what life has in store down the line. Is it possible that someone else in my life will need my kidney in twenty years from now? Is it possible that I might need it for myself? Perhaps. However, it is equally possible, that nobody will ever need my kidney and holding onto it "just in case" could prove to be a waste.

Perhaps the person who decides to keep their kidney for a rainy day will live a long and uneventful life, die an old man and be lovingly buried in the earth with two kidneys - neither of which were ever used to save anyone's life. Alternatively, one can be cut down in the prime of life simply by stepping off the curb into the path of an oncoming bus - losing not only his own life, but the additional kidney, which was a lifeline to save another person.

In my mind, this decision is akin to a person who is out on a boat, wearing a life-jacket and enjoying a beautiful day. As he looks out into the water, he sees a struggling swimmer, thrashing and gasping to breathe. However, rather than take off his own life-jacket and throw it to the drowning victim, he weighs the decision and concludes that he would rather keep the life-jacket for himself just in case he ever ends up in the water and needs help swimming. After all, why should he put his own life in danger, knowing that for him, keeping his life-jacket would mean the difference between life and death?

As a therapist, I am a major proponent of self-preservation and self-care. However, when a human life hangs in the balance and steps can be taken to save that drowning person, despite some risk and discomfort, my personal tendency is to take a chance and invest in the life of another person.

Even as I write these words I wonder what the future holds in store for me. If in ten years from now I died prematurely because of something related to my kidney donation, I suppose most of the world would say, "you see, he should not have donated his kidney." However, my deep personal perspective is that I am at peace with that. Personally, I would gladly forfeit my own life-jacket. I would rather live a life of meaning, even if I die in the process, know my life and my death were for a purpose, rather than live a life of fear, looking away from the drowning person whose life I could otherwise try to save.

The final decision to actually donate the kidney is a decision based on so many factors, many of which are out of one's own hands. When I began the process,

I had no idea whether or not I would go through with it, or if I was even a viable candidate for surgery. However, the personal responsibility I felt was to at least explore, research and begin the process.

At the end of the day, I wanted to know that even if I was not accepted as a candidate, I had at least done my part to offer the life-jacket to someone who needed it more than I did at that very moment in time.

99. Will I have any regrets?

There is poetic beauty in this question, as it was the ultimate question of all questions, and yet, it had no answers. One should not be fooled into thinking the answer exists, for it is impossible for anyone to know ahead of time.

The process of exploring kidney donation was not a search for cheerleaders who would encourage me and help me along the way. In fact, most medical professionals were cautious and perhaps even discouraging, because the decision was mine and they did not want to sway my thinking. The autonomy the donor must have in this process is absolutely sacred. Thus, if things go well - it was my decision to donate. Alternatively, if things did not go as hoped, I have to be able to own that reality as well.

Might a negative outcome lead one to feel regret? Certainly. But that is exactly what this exploration, education and transformation process was all about.

Are there ever any guarantees in life? A person might go through years of schooling and not find a job. One may train their entire lives to compete in the Olympics, but never qualify.

Life is measured, not by the finish line, but rather the effort we exert to get there.

How can one ever know what regrets he or she may face? It is a reality which will only be discovered when one is willing to take some risk. For me, the entire process of kidney donation was an exploration of myself, my strengths, my fears and my faith.

I always felt, that it is important for a donor to not be naïve about this endeavor. Instead, to research, understand and embrace these risks and concerns. For in the end, if one decides to move forward with the donation, he or she should do so wholeheartedly. That was my mindset.

I did not ignore the risks, nor turn a blind eye to them. Instead, I studied them, confronted them and strove to understand them. Ultimately, I came to the conclusion, that I was willing to join the ranks of those who, against all logic, run into fiery buildings to save a human life.

I was confident I had done every bit of research and homework imaginable and from a medical perspective, was comfortable with the decision I made to donate a kidney. It is true there are no guarantees in life. But, despite each of the risks I would faced, I was at peace with my choice, and with the knowledge that I had taken every possible step to be as prepared as possible.

A kidney donor is among a select group of people in the world. Much like the firefighter, police-officer, or military personnel, the donor is comfortable stepping up and putting his or herself at risk for the humble and distinct honor of helping those in need. Just as these heroic professionals rely upon their training and preparation to help get them through difficult situations, the kidney donor does the same. From a physical, mental, emotional, medical and spiritual standpoint, it was my research and preparation that gave me the ability to confront what others might call a heroic situation.

At the same time, I write these words with great trepidation and humility, knowing not everyone will have as positive an outcome as me, and in some cases, the outcome may even be catastrophic. One kidney donor described to me the three follow-up surgeries he required due to complications after his kidney donation to a total stranger. When I told him how sorry I was to hear about it, he said, "why are you sorry? I would still do it again and again every time!"

This mindset captures the magic of this transformative process. Although it is not for everyone, there is a growing number of people who see the value of giving life as larger than themselves, their own happiness, or their own comfort.

Such was my personal commitment and resolve to the sanctity of every life. I felt profoundly blessed to have an ability to relieve the suffering of one human being and give her back - not just life, but her dignity, family and future.

There was a turning point in this year-long process, when I began to feel that the only regret I would have would be to not take the steps toward saving the life of another person, whom I was blessed with the ability to save. That became the new definition of regret. It was not only a decision about surgery, but an existential decision. I did not want to live the rest of my life knowing I could have done more to save someone's life, but chose not to.

100. Would I do it again?

The answer for me, as it is with the many donors with whom I have spoken is, YES! I have consistently been inspired by the many kidney donors I have met. They see themselves humbly as part of a special secret club. It is a club for people who do not think much of their decision. They are individuals who simply feel they had something extra they were not using, so why not give it away to someone else who needs it?

While it may seem like an oversimplified attitude, this process begs the question as to how one values kindness, particularly in a society where people tend to focus largely on themselves.

All the donors I have spoken to have generally reported positive experiences. However, after hearing so many positive reports, I eventually grew skeptical. After all, how is it possible that everyone could be reporting such wonderful feelings about something so intense and potentially painful?

I then realized their positive experiences did not necessarily mean that everyone had an easy, quick or pain-free recovery. It meant they had no regrets and would do it again. It meant they value kindness and the gift of life to another person, over their own comfort.

Will there always be people who can report negative experiences? Absolutely. However, in my mind, this decision was a matter of weighing both sides carefully. Once I had gathered all of the information and filled my head with all the facts, statistics and numbers, together with my family, I was going to make the ultimate decision using my heart.

Think about whenever a person voluntarily signs up for the military. One could argue that they be committed and locked up for insanity? Why would a person willingly put life and limb on the line? The answer is, that while they would deny the title, such people are truly heroes. They have found great purpose and meaning by living for a value which is greater than any one individual.

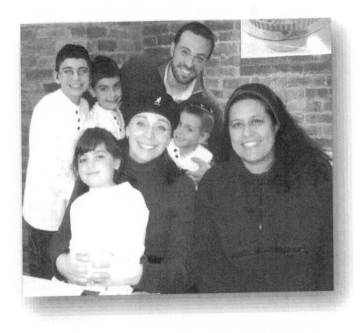

For this segment of the population, life is given greater meaning, by giving life to others. If, tragically, during that process, such heroes lose their lives, it is a risk they are willing to take, for it elevates the importance of having lived an existence that is greater than oneself. Such people contribute to the world in an elevated way. They shape and mold a society, which will continue to support and promote the notion of kindness and personal sacrifice above the individual.

As kidney donors, we do not view ourselves as heroes, or having done anything special. Rather, we simply are the ones who have stepped up to do our part to make the world and the lives of the people around us that much better.

As the Revolutionary War soldier, Nathan Hale said in his final words, "I only regret that I have but one life to give for my country," I would adapt that great slogan to say, "*I only regret that I have but one kidney to give.*" If I had the opportunity to do it all over again, I would say yes every single time.

Chapter 10.
Testimonials

The prospect of receiving a donated kidney would not just be a dream come true for myself and give me new life, but it would also help guarantee a secure and hopeful future for my family. Both my parents suffered from kidney failure and both passed away much too young. My own son has at least a 50% chance of living with Chronic Kidney Disease or End Stage Renal Failure. A donated kidney would breathe new life into those I love, and welcome us with the hope we so desperately need.

— *Cortney Smith*

Because someone gave her kidney to my husband, we can continue to give back and help others. Since then, we have become foster-parents. We now believe that, while you cannot change the whole world, you can change the whole world for one person.

— *Truus Zomer-Hille, The Netherlands*

For me, receiving a kidney meant the difference between merely existing and being able to fully participate in life.

— *Vicki, Chicago, IL*

My non-directed kidney donation in 2015 wound up saving the life of a 13-year-old boy, not only changed his life, but had profound positive ripple effects throughout his family.

When I met my recipient and his family 4 months after our surgeries, I learned his father was a single dad raising 4 boys. He was constantly tired and stressed due to worrying about and caring for his son's lifelong illness. The dialysis machine would loudly alarm and need immediate attention almost every evening, since his son would accidentally turn in his sleep while the machine was actively cleansing his body's blood through a port in his abdomen.

As they were thanking me, to help me realize just what my donation was able to stop the need for, they lifted my recipient's shirt slightly and showed me where the dialysis port used to be. My recipient was happy to tell me he could now return to school instead of learning from home, and he was now able play with his friends! He is also now able to be an active big brother with his siblings, and since the 4 months between the donation and our meeting, his father has been blessed with a new job and new wife!

My single act of love for a stranger ushered in positivity and hope to a family on the brink of despair, which in turn may have influenced every single other positive event to follow. I honestly believe we are blessed with two kidneys to allow us the joy of giving one to someone in need. I hope this helps increase awareness and inspires more people to give when so many are suffering. It is hard for me to understand why more people do not give.

— *Carrie DeLisle*

Amazingly, it was my daughter who was my donor! We adopted her when she was only two-weeks old. Thirty years later, she was my match for a kidney transplant.

She said, "you saved me, now I'm going to save you."

My medical story is ADPK - Adult Polycystic Kidney Disease. Unfortunately, it is a disease which is rampant in my family. I prayed for years that I would be able to live until my daughter was at least 18 years old. Today, she is 44 and I will soon be 75.

God had His hand in this, I truly believe. She wouldn't let anyone be tested until she did it first. She just knew she was the one!

— *Betty Lowry*

What if there was a way to eradicate End Stage Renal Disease? A way to help those now languishing on the Kidney Waiting List to get their lives back? If it sounds too good to be true, it is not. The solution to this crisis lies in Living Kidney Donation promoted via Social Media and other strategies - you can be part of this SOLUTION! Helping someone is what life is all about.

— *KidneyBuzz.com*

By donating a kidney, I did not just improve the life of one man. Rather, I gave 2 sons more time with their dad, and a wife more time with her husband. I helped keep a family together. It doesn't get better than that, does it?

— *Buffy Sexton*

As a donor and kidney matchmaker, I have seen that when someone receives a kidney, they have so much appreciation for their new lease on life. Many get their energy back, and are able to go back to work, spend more time with family and friends and are able to return to doing the things they love. Kidney recipients are so grateful to receive the gift of life and donors are blessed to be able to share that gift.

— *Chaya Lipschutz, KidneyMitzvah.com*

It is a whirlwind of emotions going through a kidney transplant, and the gift of life someone can give you is truly amazing. The sacrifice of the donor's family is something special. To give someone a second chance to live a normal life and not be dictated by dialysis is truly amazing.

— *Sam, United Kingdom*

As I am a home hemodialysis patient awaiting my 4th transplant, a healthy kidney would give me the energy to really enjoy life again!

— Brian Egerton, Manchester, UK

Getting a kidney means freedom. Being set free from prison bondage and outside to the free world again. Giving me back the opportunity to "LIVE" again. An opportunity that has been stolen away from me due to this demon of an illness/disease.

— Marcey Mighty

As an independent living organ donor advocate and president and co-founder of the American Living Organ Donor Network, I work every day to help living organ donors give the gift of life. But, I also believe society needs to do more to help donors. There are some policies in place to protect donors, but not enough. In addition to informing, supporting, and helping donors in whatever way we can with their immediate donation-related needs, the ALODN also works to change laws and regulations to be more supportive of donors. Donors should have all their donation-related expenses covered. However, if it became public policy to incentivize donors, it would diminish the moral value of what donors do and compromise the system.

The many benefits that ALODN is working to create include full medical coverage of all donation-related complications, psychological counseling, job security and coverage of lost wages. The last two benefits should also be available for the donor's care-giver who helps the donor before, during, and after surgery. Living donation is a great gift, and as a society it is our moral obligation to support donors by providing them with a medical and financial safety net, and any other benefits necessary to make the giving of that gift go as smoothly as possible. The American Living Organ Donor Network is the only 501(c)(3) organization that we know of where helping donors is our sole mission. We fully believe that taking better care of donors is a way to increase the availability of organs, but for us, donors and their needs come first.

 – *Sigrid Fry-Revere*

I am a 64-year-old woman that just donated a kidney a few weeks ago to a stranger. My recipient is now off of dialysis and will hopefully watch his children as they grow up and get married. It was a bit of a rough road for both of us, but I am so glad that I did it. My amazing husband, children and grandchildren have been so incredibly supportive. I am gratified to watch my recipient get better and stronger each day and move on with the rest of his life!

— *Cheryl, New York*

I received a kidney from my sister in 1978 in Milwaukee, WI. I am happy to report that after 38 years, I have been extremely fortunate, having experienced no rejection episodes! Thus far my sister's kidney continues to work fine!

— *Dan Holm*

Being a 2-time kidney transplant recipient and the founder of the Living Kidney Donors Network (www.LKDN.org), I am particularly moved by this book. Saving a life by being a living kidney donor is one of the most precious and powerful acts anyone can do, and Ari Sytner is one of those special individuals. As a non-directed donor, (donating even when you don't know someone who needs a kidney transplant,) Ari joins a small group of fewer than 1%

of living kidney donors. With his book, Ari is continuing his commitment to this critical need by helping educate others and inspiring future living kidney donors.

— *Harvey Mysel*

My sisters and I know firsthand, just how invaluable and amazing altruistic living kidney donation is. We saw this after our father's life was saved by a complete stranger. Through our kidney foundation we see each and every day, how lives are forever changed by altruistic donors. Love. Give. Life - Flood Sisters Kidney Foundation www.Floodsisters.org

— *Jennifer, Cynthia & Heather Flood*

Thank you to the following sponsors who, among MANY other kind-hearted people from around the world, generously stepped up to support the publication of this book:

Austec Business Transitions, LLC.

Yosi Applebaum

Albert Behar

Rachel and Mordy Book

Ann Marie Brunk

Jacob R. Burke

CZ

Cheryl and Eddie Dauber

Allan Dougramachi

Shlomo Fried

Glenna Baumbarger Frey

Linda K. Trestman and David M. Gilston

Stuart M. Greenstein, MD

Aaron and Adina Halpert

William Hochman

Lea Hanan

Jason E. Huff

Carrie Idler & Family

Moshe & Devora Isenberg and Family

Christine Kerravala

Garry Kravit

Terry & Betty Lowry

Lynn A. Polizzi, LCSW

Elke & Mordechai Pollak

The Nirenblatt Family

Mark Skovron & Jeff Peltin

Yossi & Gitty Preiserowicz

Devora Ratner

Nathan and Judy Rephan

Mendy Reiner

Debra and Miles Rosen

Seth

Freida and Joe Sokol

Barry & Betty Sytner

Sharon Sytner (aka Mom)

Rabbi Tzvi Sytner

Marc Wohlgemuth & Associates P.C.

Jonathan Z.

Jessica and Jeffrey Zucker

A letter from Ronit:

It makes me so happy that Ari has written about his experience as a kidney donor. By doing so, he shows the world that it is important to help other people who cannot go on with life. As they look out at the possibility of death, it becomes very difficult to really live life. Yet, what Ari has done for me, truly shows what a special person he is, in so many ways! To give a part of your own body is not a common thing to do, and it is quite remarkable.

From the first time I met Ari, I knew that he was unique. It was a few days before the surgery took place, and I remember how he thanked ME for giving him the opportunity to save a life.

When we were in the pre-op room, waiting to be called to the surgery room, Ari was called to go first. Yet, before he went, he came over to me and gave me his blessing. It was not just a simple "good luck," but it was a deep, heartfelt and real prayer.

Since the transplant we are in touch at least once a week, every Friday, for saying Shabbat Shalom, and I am grateful to him for that. My family and I were very honored and excited when Ari and his wonderful family invited us to attend his son's Bar-Mitzvah celebration, which recently took place in Israel. The entire reunion was very emotional for all of us. As I now prepare to marry off my first daughter, I hope that we will continue to celebrate all of life's joys and milestones together, as he is part of the family!

Thank you Ari — and again, 'Thank You' is only a simple gesture, because your gift truly gave me my life back.

Love,
Ronit

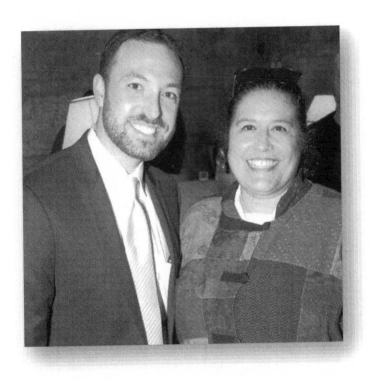

Kindness -

Although it is not always easy and often comes with sacrifice, it is the small price we pay to give our children and society a far better world.

Please feel free to contact Ari for speaking engagements, book-signing events, consultations, coaching, partnerships or questions.

www.asytner.com
@arisytner on Twitter
ari@asytner.com

66602752R00123

Made in the USA
Middletown, DE
13 March 2018